Fat Loss Without Dieting

Revised 2020

With NEW Content!

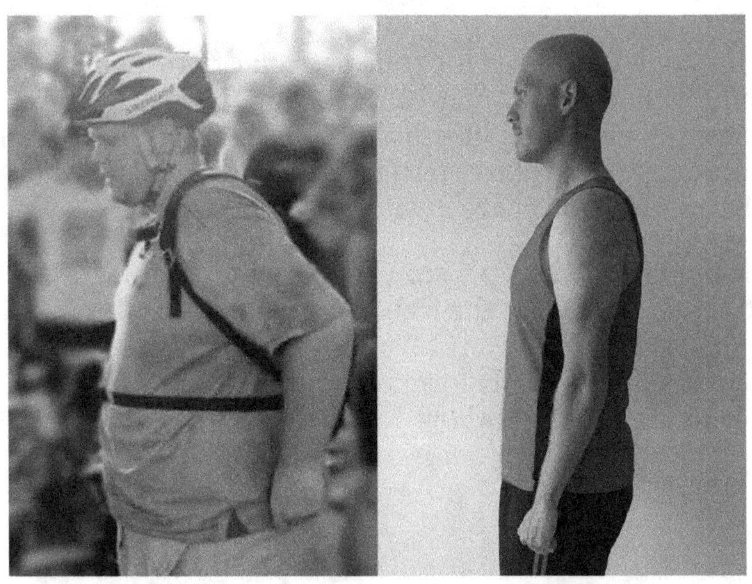

Stop starving. Stop counting calories.
Stop overexericising, and start losing weight!

By Craig Roberts

Table of contents

Table of Contents

Introduction

Thank you

First of all, thank you from the bottom of my heart for buying this book. I thank you for two reasons, reason one, because you, buying this makes me so happy that another person has found the information I have, which helped me to lose over 140lbs and change my life completely. Two, because I would like to thank you for believing in me, at least having the slightest bit of faith that the information I provide can help you. I'm happy that you've found this book and I really hope you can use this information to change your life, just as I did.

Who is this book for?

Anyone wanting to lose weight in a safe, steady and consistent manner. You won't find any "6 pack abs in 6 weeks" or "bikini body guides" here. If you're someone who wants to lose weight and has tried the gimmicks, the starvation, the restriction and are still not at your goal size/weight as you read this, then this book is for you.

Maybe you've tried "low carb" diets or simply restricting your calories only to find yourself starving at the end of the day and going for those fatty, sugary refined junk foods. I've been there and done that I can assure you, I've tried calorie restriction, low carb diets and even special military diets and all have left me starving, low energy, and caving into all the wrong foods, (despite my strong will power). One of those diets even had me almost black out while I was working a relatively manual job as a 15-year-old boy... despite normally having boundless energy, (more on this later)!

What to expect from this book?

First of all, I'm a very no nonsense guy, this book WON'T be filled with "fluff" just to fill pages and word counts, I will outline and compact all of the information I have on losing weight, but more importantly, losing FAT, (more on this later), in an efficient and effective manner, in as few words and pages as possible. During a lot of this book it will be like I'm talking to you in person and we're having a face to face conversation, one without all the hairs and graces that you might expect from an "Atkins diet" or "low carb" diet styled book. But never the less it will be informative and give you the tools to go out there and start or continue your weight loss journey but this time heading in the RIGHT direction! Each chapter, of which there will be many will be dedicated to a certain topic and I will cover in a much detail as you need, feel free to highlight sentences, take notes etc. as you're going along. Some of this book you may need to re-read many times for it to sink in, or some of it you may want to keep coming back to as reference.

For those of you who have seen me on YouTube or other social media you may know me as: Craig's Transformation, Cycling Slimmer, Cycling Slim or even Carbedupvegan. The rest of you can just call me Craig Roberts.

The heaviest weight I saw on the scales was 310lbs but at points I could have been 10-30lbs heavier as I didn't start weighing myself until weeks into my new lifestyle as I was too scared to accept reality! I don't often weigh myself now as I'm currently in the muscle building/toning phase, but the last time I did the scales sat at around 168lbs.

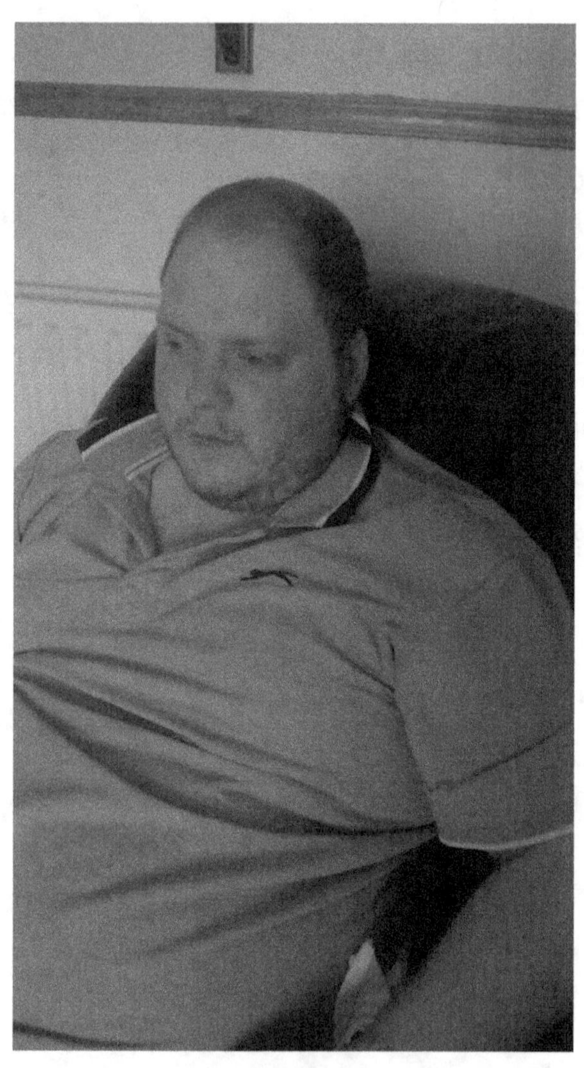

Me in 2014

Chapter 1 – Who am I to write this book?

Who I was and who I am now?

When I first started my weight loss journey, I was over 310lbs, struggled to walk 200m to the local convenience store for cigarettes or alcohol and certainly wasn't a "fan of exercise". I would spend my days lounging on my lazy boy sofa, surfing the internet and playing video games until 6am in the morning, getting up at 2-4pm, (sometimes in winter waking up in the dark!) I was unemployed and basically unemployable due to my downright laziness, and would break a sweat just sitting in my chair.

How did I let myself get like this you might ask? DEPRESSION. It is a simple word to a much more complex problem but for now that word will suffice. I was in a vicious circle where I was extremely unhappy with my size and weight and current life so I would binge eat, binge drink, and basically take my mind off my issues via video games, TV shows and movies. I managed to limit my excessive alcohol consumption of which I would easily drink 1-2 bottles of wine as a "starter" then I'd move onto the "main course" of usually, Jack Daniels and coke, to which I'd drink around 500ml of the whiskey with as much coke as was needed and yet I still wouldn't get drunk, that's how adapted I had become. I nevertheless felt somewhat calmer and more relaxed and it allowed me to forget about my problems for that night. Accompanying that I would have takeout food, usually greasy kebabs, burgers, pizzas and snacks, both salty and sweet. Of course I made a few feeble attempts at weight loss which usually involved calorie restriction, (more on this later), all of which failed within a week or so and I'd have a heavy refeeding period where I'd binge out on anything and everything but the kitchen sink, and no doubt gain back the weight I'd lost plus interest! I also tried to exercise and back in 2013 I even refurbished an old bike I had in the shed, did a few rides with, and planned to tour around Europe with. I boarded a ferry from Hull in England to Bruges, Belgium, I managed to cycle around 5km before contacting my friend via free WIFI to collect me in his very small hatchback. He took me to his house and I stayed there for around 5 days which most of the time was spent playing video games, drinking beer and eating pizza before he got sick of me lazing around and insisted, I left. Then with all my belongings on a ridiculously heavy trailer I then cycled 2km to a nearby campsite and stayed there for 2 more days. I spoke with my parents and was very emotional, I'd never been away from home this long and I felt lost, lonely and missed home. We decided it was best for me to come home and I took the next available ferry and left... so much for my big tour around Europe!

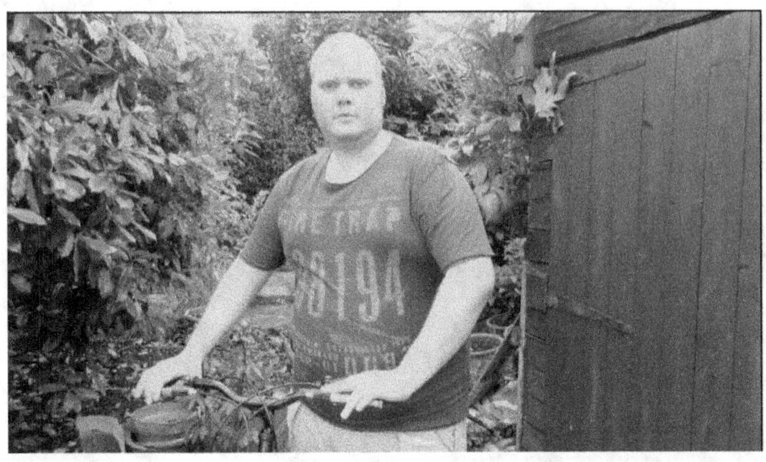

I could go on all day about many instances of my laziness or lack of fitness such as the time I went to a local motor racing track to see the cars and spent literally the whole day moaning to my friend that I wanted to sit down, or the time I rode less than 2km at a slow pace on my bike and got home and literally had an asthma attack but I think you get the message of how big and unfit I was...

Now I'm around 175lbs depending on the time of day, how much I've eaten, drank, (more on this later.) I am certainly no stranger to exercise. Participating in 5-6 days a week MINIMUM, and it doesn't feel like a chore whatsoever, it's literally a part of my life now. Nobody forces me to, and I certainly don't have some drill sergeant style character shouting at me to get out of the door each day. So, what's changed? How did I go from the above-mentioned lazy person, to someone who thinks nothing of cycling up a mountain, or riding

100km (fueled) before breakfast? This you'll find out in later chapters, what clicked to make me change and more importantly what made me want to change.

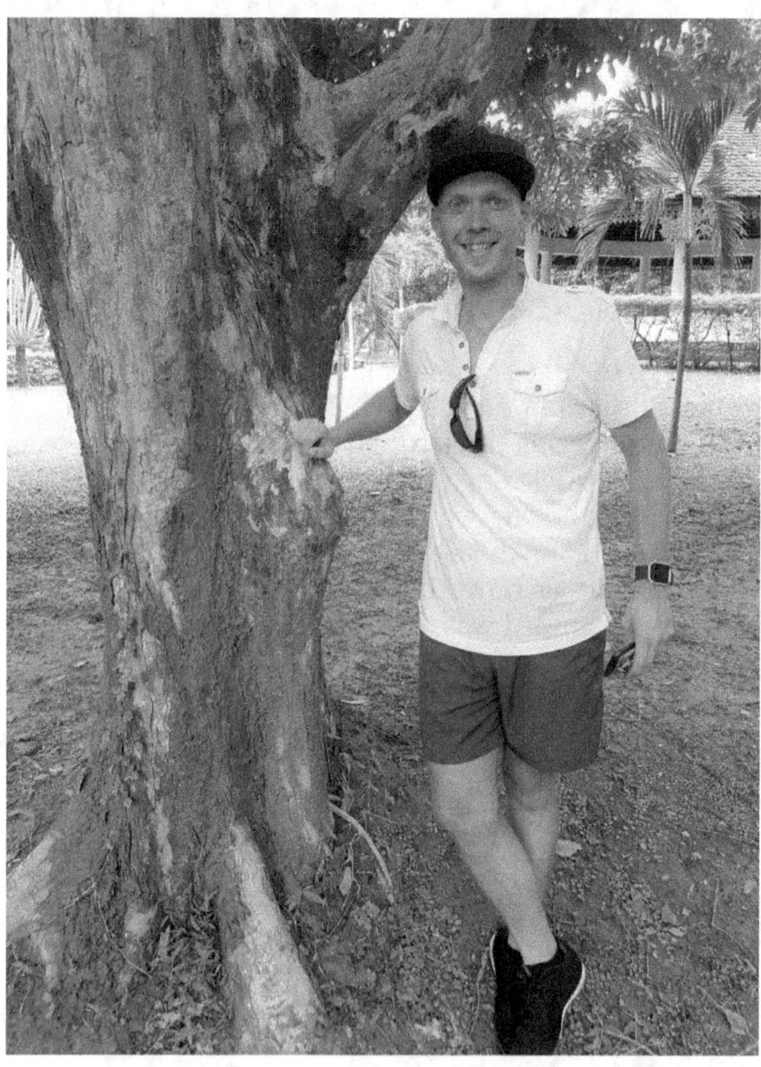

So, I'm NOT a qualified health professional, I don't have a piece of paper and I haven't spent 3+ years at university learning the kind of bad nutrition and exercise advice which keep people obese anyway. Does it matter? In my opinion NO, real world experience is what really matters, sure people may have a shiny certificate or been preached to by some preppy ivy league college but often the people who have these qualifications make books like the "Atkin's Diet" anyway, and people are still not just fat but getting FATTER! A great example of this; the Belgium Minister of Social Affairs and Health in the Michel Government is a morbidly obese woman. She is hardly at all a role model for health despite having the credentials.

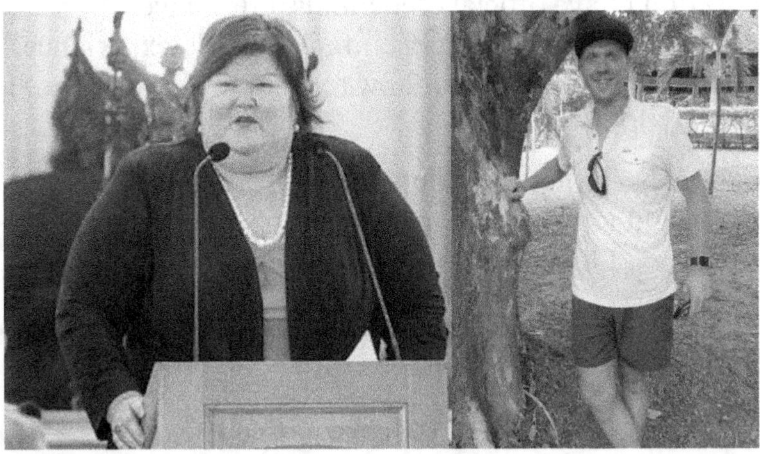

Who would you rather take weight loss advice from? YET I'm not qualified, but she is, do you see where I'm going with this? I've tried it all and really found what works for me and many others, I've even coached many others to losing weight.

Who am I to write this book?

To ask the question again, I think I'm someone who has been there and done that and helped others do the same. I haven't just read about it or theorized it. It wasn't easy but it also wasn't as hard as I expected. So, stick with me as I guide you through your weight loss journey.

Chapter 1 Conclusion

- I came from an obese, lazy background, and went from 310lbs to around 168lbs.

- I don't have official credentials, but I have something more important. Real world experience, and the knowledge of how to lose weight, for myself and others.

- I've been there and done that, with regards to weight loss, and I don't have a shady back story... nor do I take steroids.

Chapter 2 – Weight loss vs fat loss

The scales don't mean everything

One of the most common terms that is thrown around in the "weight loss industry" (notice weight loss) is "losing weight", or I've lost xx amount of lbs. Many diet books or plans will promise that you'll lose 7lbs in 1 week or you'll lose 14 lbs in 1 month and they are not lying when they say "weight" either. But the most important thing you should be setting out to lose is FAT. Sure, you can be following the "standard American diet", eating your unhealthy meals each day with unhealthy snacks. Drinking alcohol to wash down your pepperoni pizza and then switch things up dramatically over a 7-day period and lose 7lbs. Often what you're doing in this time is losing water weight, it would be very hard to lose 7lbs of pure fat in 7 days, which is 24,500 calories or around 3500 calories each day. I doubt Chris Froome during the Tour de France would burn much more than that each day! Another thing I will add here is take into account muscle mass, for example if you are gaining muscle, don't expect the scales to still read the same, they may even go up. I went through a stage where I just started lifting weights and despite looking trimmer each week as I was getting rid of fat and gaining muscle, my weight stayed the same. Some weeks it even went up! At this point on my journey I decided it wasn't practical to weigh myself anymore.

Which is more important to lose?

It sounds like a silly question but it really depends on where you are with your current body, some people may be 7lbs overweight but not be fat at all and could just be carrying around excess food in the guts, (more on this later), and excess water retention due to too much sodium, and not enough sweating from exercise. Then on the other hand there could be the otherwise healthy person who is carrying 7lbs excess pure fat on them but doesn't eat much salt and exercises regularly. So, everyone has different goals but I am guessing if you're reading this book, you have a little more than 7lbs to lose. Excess fat is the most important thing to remove from your body, more so than water even as holding water isn't actually bad for the body, it's more of an annoyance and can be quickly dealt with unlike fat. Now I will never say to aim for a certain weight or you should weigh as much as somebody else. Everybody is different and each person has different muscle mass, bone mass etc.

How weight fluctuations can be normal

So you weigh yourself on a Monday morning at 7am just after a bowel movement and you are, let's say 200.2lbs. That's great, maybe your down 2lbs from last week. You weigh yourself Wednesday morning at the same time, also after a bowel movement, and your 201.5lbs, OH NO YOU'VE GAINED WEIGHT! The reality is your body may have a bit more food going through the digestive system, you may have more water being stored, or if you're a female you could be holding excess water due to a menstrual cycle approaching. Not to mention maybe the day you were lighter you exercised more and therefore used up more fluids, more glycogen. The bottom line here is; if you're going to use the scales, use them over a period of time. I would suggest weekly or monthly weigh ins, and keep a graph style progress chart. Be sure to weigh in under the same conditions too. It's no good weighing in on a morning before breakfast and fluids one week, then the next week weighing in just after dinner as you could have gained 5lbs or more throughout the day on food and fluids. If you have followed this advice but gained up to 5lbs, ask yourself why? Did you have a sodium packed weekend, did you exercise less this week, all these things can really fluctuate your weight so don't worry.

Keep progress pictures

As the saying goes, "a picture is worth a thousand words", and that is so true also for your journey of fat loss. Sometimes, especially if your gaining muscle, whether by weight lifting or just toning through cardio, such as cycling or running, you can be slimming down but gaining or staying the same weight. This can be so off putting for people who are a slave to the scales. Meanwhile their friends and family may be commenting on their new slim physique. I personally have kept progress pictures over my journey, (not as many as I would like), but that is how you really see the changes, even if the scales are giving you bad readings. Monthly, or maybe even weekly progress photos, could be a great way to watch the fat strip away and see those muscle gains and could be an inspiration for friends or family to also slim down. So don't be a slave to the scales, but be sure to use them as an objective way of keeping progress over time.

Chapter 2 Conclusion

- Your weight will fluctuate during the day *and* over time, so don't rely 100% on the scales, it might not give an accurate reading.

- Use the scales as a baseline over a period of months to observe a downward pattern.

- It's more important to lose fat than water.

- Take pictures as well as weighing yourself.

- The number on the scales doesn't mean anything, DON'T let it define you!

Chapter 3 – Why you shouldn't "Diet"

Lose weight quickly diets

If you're reading this book, you're no stranger to the typical fad diets, where in theory you can lose 7lbs in a week or get ripped six pack abs in 6 weeks, but then what? What do you do after the 7 days is up or the 6 weeks, you put all of the weight back on PLUS interest! Why is this? Well by calorie restricting your body can lose weight quickly initially by being shocked into dipping into excess fat stores and by usually consuming more water and water rich foods combined with exercise. Usually your body will quickly adapt though, and slow down your metabolic rate so that you can't lose weight too quickly or even any more doing what you're currently doing, (more on this later). Not long after this point you hit a plateau and lose interest causing you to binge out or fall back into your old ways, this simple cycle makes the weight loss and fitness industry billions! I've tried so many of these diets in the past. I remember doing a diet when I was 15; I ate eggs, low calorie fruits, and vegetables. This diet was the one I mentioned above. I was working at a fruit and vegetable store at the time and doing manual labor before and after school. Anyway, I'd been on this diet for 2 days and I went to work in the morning to do my usual 2-hour shift, only to nearly pass out whilst lifting a box of bananas. My boss at the time came over and told me to sit down on the bench and he swiftly brought me some ripe bananas which I gorged on and immediately felt better, never again I had thought! That certainly wasn't the last time I'd use the wrong, but conventional, way to lose weight, and end up starving, miserable, and back where I started.

Why these "get results quickly" style diets are flawed

Any kind of way of eating and or exercising that you can only sustain for a 1-12-week period is NOT a sustainable way of life. Ask yourself this: Can I do this diet/exercise plan for the rest of my life without it feeling starving and/or excessively tired? If you answered no, then I'm guessing that's why you're reading this book. What usually happens is you start a plan like this, eager and full of excitement, you lose some weight and then comes the crash, either you feel so starving and tired that you give into "bad foods" again, or you just lose interest because you're not seeing results anymore. Either way, you can't go on like this, you need to get on a plan for life. Many of you have watched the TV show "The biggest loser" I'm sure. You see the contestant's work their asses off and lose crazy amounts of weight, in short periods of time. But then what happens? You may not hear of that person again, or if you do they've usually gained all the weight back, or at least gone back to their old habits. This is what the industry feeds on. If you simply went to your doctor or diet specialist, and they laid exactly what you needed to do to get healthy and stay healthy for the rest of your life, they'd all be out of business and you certainly wouldn't want or need to go back.

Chapter 3 Conclusion

- Most of the weight loss of "lose weight quickly" diets, come from water weight, NOT fat.

- In time, "diets" will slow your down your metabolism.

- "Diets" are NOT sustainable for life.

- You'll end up gaining the weight back and extra!

Chapter 4 – Lose the perfectionist mindset

I could honestly fill up a whole book on this topic, some even have. But I'm trying to cut the point here, nobody in the history of humans was ever perfect, no matter how they may have seemed on the surface. In the real world there can often be no success with at least some failure. Athletes for example, don't start their first race as a winner (usually), they have to lose many, many times, before they get their first win and that's usually what helps drive them to in the first place. Often today's billionaires would have failed many, many times, only to get back up again stronger and wiser for it. Sure, when you have actually heard of these people, they may on the surface seem perfect because they've been there and done that with the making silly mistakes. They will however make good mistakes but they just have a good PR crew to help clean up those messes and keep them from the public eye and to avoid stock crashes! Usually we can learn from our mistakes and that is what makes us grow as people and learn. Failure isn't a bad thing, it's just part of succeeding! One thing that people can end up doing is focusing too much on perfection and that can be both a blessing and curse. It's good to take pride in the way you do things and to try to do things correctly, but to take things to extremes and aim for perfection every time can be a real drag. I should know, this was the kind of mentality I had and it really did me no good in the long run. It caused me a lot of negative feelings when I stepped on the scales when I hadn't lost enough weight, or I hadn't lost any at all. These feelings would often ruin my day, or lead me on a downward spiral... Often binging out on bad foods due to my emotional state, (nothing to do with wrong diet etc.). Often as well, people with this kind of mindset will have a "go big or go home" mentality and if they can't ride 2 hours on the bike, they will do nothing, or feel like they've failed. When reality is doing 1 hour even, just getting out the door is something to be proud of! We all have off days no matter who you are and how fit or determined you are, but we have to be kind to ourselves and not punish ourselves for not being perfect, nobody is!

Just do the best you can

All you can promise yourself each day when you wake up is to do the best you can with what you're given or have at that moment in time, no more, no less. If you give it your best, you give it 100%, you can't do any better than that and you should, no matter what you've achieved (or not), be proud of yourself. Know that you did all you could.

Remove the all-or-nothing mindset

The all or nothing mindset won't get you anywhere, these people will often see things as "black or white" or they will "fail or succeed". There is no in-between, or grey area. Most importantly though, love and respect yourself enough to not punish yourself for every mistake you make. Be kind enough to give yourself the chance to get up and try again, this time stronger and wiser.

Chapter 4 Conclusion

- Many professional athletes and billionaires all started making mistakes to get where they are today.

- Failure isn't a bad thing.

- All you have to do is give 100%, no more, no less, and you can go away feeling satisfied.

- Remove the "all or nothing" mindset.

Chapter 5 – Stop comparing yourself to others

Are celebrities really good role models to aspire to?

Most people look to a so-called celebrity's body in magazines or in films and think that is how they should look, or "I want that body". With the few exceptions most celebrities are very slim during filming, and photo shoots especially. So that's how you perceive them. What you don't see however is what a lot of them are doing behind the scenes to get like that. Usually before a role or a photo shoot comes up, they will fad diet, (as I mentioned in Chapter 3). As soon as the role is finished, or the photo shoot is complete, they binge out and go on holiday and usually you see them in the paper on a beach having ballooned out, gaining 5-10+kgs and looking unhealthy. The fact of the matter is, they don't live a sustainable lifestyle and you shouldn't aspire to be like this. It's the same with a lot of male actors you see in the movies, suddenly you see them get very muscular for a role within a short time period such as 6 months (usually for a super hero role), and the man on the street thinks he can imitate that with a few protein shakes and a few months at the gym. Generally, the actors will be taking steroids under the doctor's supervision to get like this for practicality reasons, maybe in another 6 months they have to lose all the muscle and play an anorexic role or it could be the other way round. A well-known actor to go through this rapid transformation is Christian Bale. For the role of The Machinist, he slimmed down to a very unhealthy, and low body fat percentage. Then just over 6 months later he bulked up, and went from around 120lbs to 220lbs. But then was told he was too big so slimmed back down by another 35lbs before his role of batman see image below.

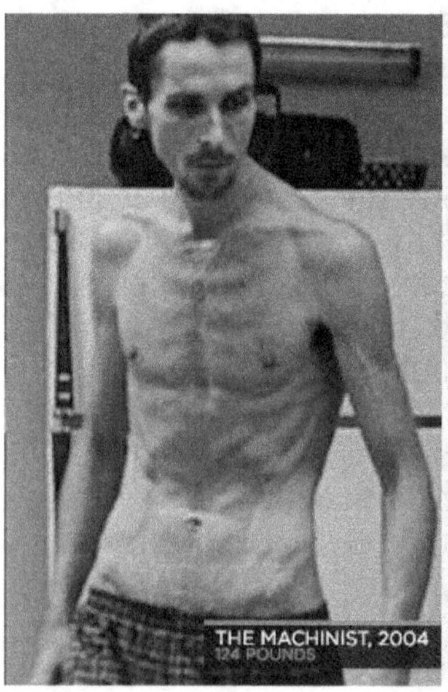

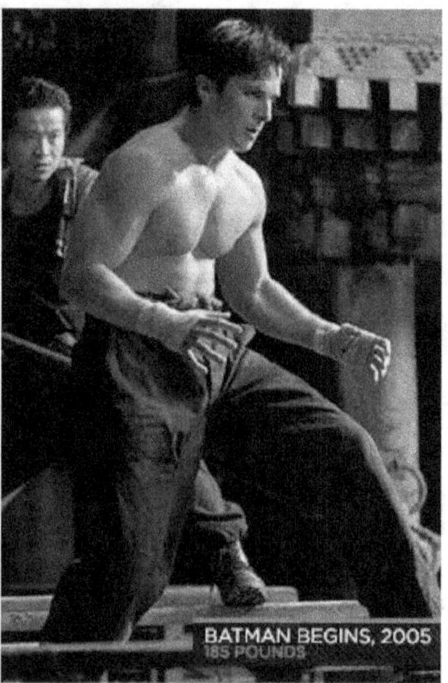

Credit to www.bodybuilding.com

So could he of done this transformation without steroids? Maybe if he was a freak of nature. But likely he wouldn't want or need to as he's not trying to be some fully natural body builder and he would take "healthy" doses under a strict doctor's supervision. What I'm trying to say here is; what you see the celebs doing, the weight loss and their shapes are not as easily obtainable by the rest of the population. So don't think it's normal to fluctuate like the celebrities do. It's more important to have a good, healthy body size and shape all year long. No cutting or bulking should be required for the average person.

Everyone is unique

Many people, (especially girls), will look at another person's figure and think "I want to look like them". I've even had clients tell me they want to look like a certain person they know of. I will tell you the same thing I told them. YOU are YOU. You can only look like YOU. You may find this off putting (they often do), but if you are overweight the best thing you can do is slim down and try to look like a less overweight version of yourself. If you have pictures of yourself when you were at your slimmest then aspire to look like that, because that's your body shape. Every person has different body shapes, and will hold healthy fat in different areas. Some people may hold fat on their butt or their stomach area, and those might be the areas they find the hardest to lose. For me personally it's the hips area. Sometimes people will have a slim person in mind that is unattainable for them personally, so it can be very disheartening to never be able to achieve that. For example, some girls have large hip bones so they have the "curvy" look, whereas other girls have a straight waist. If you have large hip bones it would be impractical for you to aspire to have a straight waist and trying to get to that could cause you to lose too much fat and get to an unhealthy body fat percentage. Which could also give you negative long-term health effects, such as loss of period, and hormonal imbalances. It's the same with guys, some men naturally gain muscle quicker and have broader shoulders so to aspire to them if you don't have those genetics is unwise. So, don't worry about what other people look like, just focus on looking the best version of yourself and aspire to that daily. For sure use others body's as inspiration, but remember you will look different which is neither a good or bad thing. We are all unique and that is a beautiful thing. There is nothing to hide or be ashamed of. Who wants to look like a cookie cutter clone of someone else? Certainly not me!

Chapter 5 Conclusion

- Stop aspiring to be like celebrities. Their bodies and physiques aren't attainable without surgery, steroids, or crash diets.

- Everybody is unique and has their own natural figures. Stop trying to look like somebody else's figure.

- Often celebrity transformations are not natural! Such as Christian bale's extreme weight loss and muscle gain in such a short period of time.

Chapter 6 – What's the best diet for humans?

Have you been lied to?

I'd say everybody at some point has heard of the "Paleo Diet". A diet in which the guidelines are pretty simple, "if a caveman didn't eat it, neither should you". When you're following the Paleo Diet, you can eat anything we could hunt or gather way back in the day – things like meats, fish, nuts, leafy greens, regional veggies, and seeds. It is evident that many of the foods we eat today are refined and processed very heavily almost beyond recognition. So, the Paleo guidelines are pretty much spot on in getting us back to our natural roots. But here lies the problem with those guidelines; it is theorized that we are "omnivores", mainly because meat is so prevalent in our lives, you see hamburger restaurants on almost every corner nowadays and almost every meal we have available contains some form of meat. There is a lot of money made in the animal agricultural business, and should overnight people suddenly stop eating meat, then all hell would break loose literally! There would be millions or maybe even billions of animals due for slaughter sent back out into the wild, the economy would crash due to many stores and restaurants reliance on meat sales. So, in schools and universities we are taught that we are omnivores so we can continue consuming meat but in a healthier fashion, with added vegetables and nuts and seeds vs hamburgers with bread and cheese. Combine the fact that consumption of animal products is the leading cause of heart disease and cancer, making big money for the pharmaceutical industry. Much more on this in books such as "The China Study" and "How Not to Die".

Where's the proof?

Have you ever looked at a live animal and thought "hmm I'd love to go up to that creature and bite a chunk out of it" ... or have you ever considered eating your pet when the cupboards were empty? And if not, ask yourself why? Have you ever walked down the meat isle in a grocery store and had the urge to eat the meat raw? Do you think without weapons, using only your nails and teeth, you could run after and kill a cow or a deer? These are typically questions you wouldn't think to ask yourself. In modern day, meat is so simple and easy to acquire, it's wrapped in a nice neat package in a safe supermarket. You can just wave a piece of plastic in front of a computer, which sends the necessary resources needed to purchase the item to the shop. You then go home, usually in some form of motorized transport, turn on your electric or gas oven or stove and cook the meat, add sauces, spices and condiments and serve it. Cavemen certainly didn't do this. The animals in the slaughter houses are hidden far from the public eyes. Meats are given different names from the animals to confuse us such as "beef", "pork", "ham", and "bacon". Chances are if you walked into a butcher and he had a live pig and you asked for some bacon and he proceeded to slaughter it before your very eyes, that bacon wouldn't seem so appealing. This book isn't here to try and convert you to a plant-based lifestyle, or to push some ideals on you. This section is to make you think. Chances are if you are reading this you've tried the conventional hamster wheel and not succeeded anyway. So, any fans of meat who might use the example of lions eating meat to justify their daily bacon sandwich, would be very wrong as I mentioned above.

Human physiology – what are we designed to eat

Although many humans choose to eat a wide variety of plant and animal foods, earning us the dubious title of "omnivore," we're anatomically frugivorous.

Teeth, Jaws, and Nails:

Humans have short, soft fingernails and pathetically small "canine" teeth. In contrast, carnivores all have sharp claws and large canine teeth that are capable of tearing flesh.

Carnivores' jaws move only up and down, requiring them to tear chunks of flesh from their prey and swallow them whole. Humans and other herbivores can move their jaws up and down and from side to side, allowing them to grind up fruit and vegetables with their back teeth. Like other herbivores' teeth, humans' back molars are flat for grinding fibrous plant foods. Carnivores lack these flat molars.

Dr. Richard Leakey, a renowned anthropologist, summarizes, "You can't tear flesh by hand, you can't tear hide by hand. Our anterior teeth are not suited for tearing flesh or hide. We don't have large canine teeth, and we wouldn't have been able to deal with food sources that require those large canines."

Stomach Acidity:

Carnivores swallow their food whole, relying on their extremely acidic stomach juices to break down flesh and kill the dangerous bacteria in meat that would otherwise sicken or kill them. Our stomach acids are much weaker in comparison, because strong acids aren't needed to digest pre-chewed fruits and vegetables.

Intestinal Length:

Carnivores have short intestinal tracts and colons that allow meat to pass through the animal relatively quickly, before it can rot and cause illness. Humans' intestinal tracts are much longer than those of carnivores of comparable size. Longer intestines allow the body more time to break down fiber and absorb the nutrients from plant-based foods, but they make it dangerous for humans to eat meat. The bacteria in meat have extra time to multiply during the long trip through the digestive system, increasing the risk of food poisoning. Meat actually begins to rot while it makes its way through human intestines, which increases the risk of colon cancer. Credit www.peta.org

Below is a chart which outlines the differences.

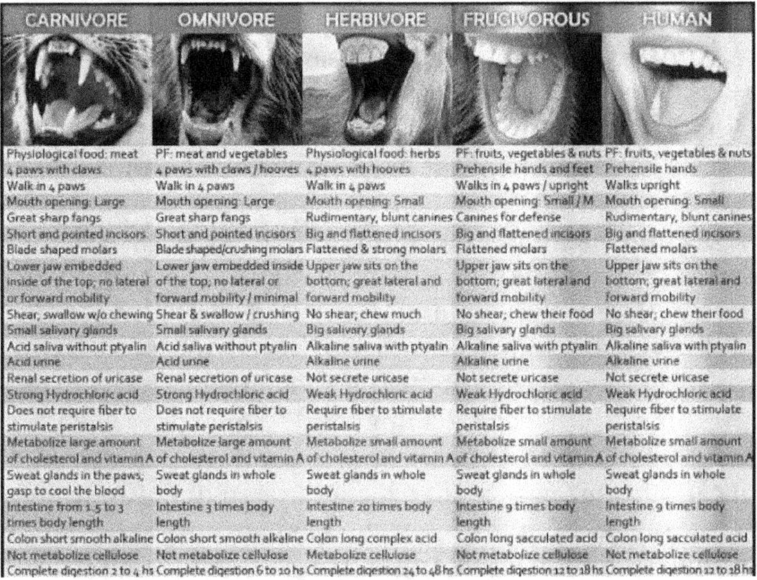

CARNIVORE	OMNIVORE	HERBIVORE	FRUGIVOROUS	HUMAN
Physiological food: meat	PF: meat and vegetables	Physiological food: herbs	PF: fruits, vegetables & nuts	PF: fruits, vegetables & nuts
4 paws with claws	4 paws with claws / hooves	4 paws with hooves	Prehensile hands and feet	Prehensile hands
Walk in 4 paws	Walk in 4 paws	Walk in 4 paws	Walks in 4 paws / upright	Walks upright
Mouth opening: Large	Mouth opening: Large	Mouth opening: Small	Mouth opening: Small / M	Mouth opening: Small
Great sharp fangs	Great sharp fangs	Rudimentary, blunt canines	Canines for defense	Rudimentary, blunt canines
Short and pointed incisors	Short and pointed incisors	Big and flattened incisors	Big and flattened incisors	Big and flattened incisors
Blade shaped molars	Blade shaped/crushing molars	Flattened & strong molars	Flattened molars	Flattened molars
Lower jaw embedded inside of the top; no lateral or forward mobility	Lower jaw embedded inside of the top; no lateral or forward mobility / minimal	Upper jaw sits on the bottom; great lateral and forward mobility	Upper jaw sits on the bottom; great lateral and forward mobility	Upper jaw sits on the bottom; great lateral and forward mobility
Shear, swallow w/o chewing	Shear & swallow / crushing	No shear, chew much	No shear; chew their food	No shear; chew their food
Small salivary glands	Small salivary glands	Big salivary glands	Big salivary glands	Big salivary glands
Acid saliva without ptyalin	Acid saliva without ptyalin	Alkaline saliva with ptyalin	Alkaline saliva with ptyalin	Alkaline saliva with ptyalin
Acid urine	Acid urine	Alkaline urine	Alkaline urine	Alkaline urine
Renal secretion of uricase	Renal secretion of uricase	Not secrete uricase	Not secrete uricase	Not secrete uricase
Strong Hydrochloric acid	Strong Hydrochloric acid	Weak Hydrochloric acid	Weak Hydrochloric acid	Weak Hydrochloric acid
Does not require fiber to stimulate peristalsis	Does not require fiber to stimulate peristalsis	Require fiber to stimulate peristalsis	Require fiber to stimulate peristalsis	Require fiber to stimulate peristalsis
Metabolize large amount of cholesterol and vitamin A	Metabolize large amount of cholesterol and vitamin A	Metabolize small amount of cholesterol and vitamin A	Metabolize small amount of cholesterol and vitamin A	Metabolize small amount of cholesterol and vitamin A
Sweat glands in the paws; gasp to cool the blood	Sweat glands in whole body	Sweat glands in whole body	Sweat glands in whole body	Sweat glands in whole body
Intestine from 1.5 to 3 times body length	Intestine 3 times body length	Intestine 20 times body length	Intestine 9 times body length	Intestine 9 times body length
Colon short smooth alkaline	Colon short smooth alkaline	Colon long complex acid	Colon long sacculated acid	Colon long sacculated acid
Not metabolize cellulose	Not metabolize cellulose	Metabolize cellulose	Not metabolize cellulose	Not metabolize cellulose
Complete digestion 2 to 4 hs	Complete digestion 6 to 10 hs	Complete digestion 24 to 48 hs	Complete digestion 12 to 18 hs	Complete digestion 12 to 18 hs

As you can see in the chart, the natural meat eaters look totally different to our physiology, this is also the same reason that eating meat and foods which we were not designed for is damaging to our health. Our bodies are not designed to eat meat and we will have adverse reactions to it, whether that be weight gain, cancer or heart disease. The same way that if you fed a carnivore vegetables and fruits, their bodies would have an adverse reaction to that as well.

So as you can see we were designed to eat vegetables, fruits, nuts, basically anything that grows from the ground we can eat, (with exceptions of course). In modern day there are mass production of other products such as cow's milk which you find in almost everything from pasta sauces, to some breads, and even candy. In nature we were designed to consume milk for a few years up until weaning, and then we would develop a lactose intolerance naturally. We certainly wouldn't go and drink another creature's milk. The same way that having sex with another creature is disgusting... could you imagine going up to a cow and sucking on its udders? The paleo diet also doesn't allow milk as we wouldn't consume it in nature. There are so many ill side effects to drinking milk. The hormones in milk are designed for baby cows and gives them just what they need to bulk up as a young calf to become a huge fully grown cow. As I mentioned earlier most people are naturally lactose intolerant but maybe they haven't been diagnosed. It can show up in many ways such as Asthma, acne, and even various cancers. Milk contains Insulin-like growth factor (IGF-1), which is a natural human growth hormone instrumental in normal growth during childhood. But in adulthood can promote abnormal growth—the proliferation, spread (metastasis), an invasion of cancer.
So, consider filling your meals full of starches, grains, vegetables, fruits, legumes, nuts and seeds. And cut out the meat, dairy, eggs and processed foods!

Chapter 6 Conclusion

- We are NOT omnivores!

- We don't find animal meat attractive, unless it's cooked and/or seasoned.

- We lack the ability to kill and eat animals using only our nails and teeth.

- Our stomach acid is too weak to digest meat, causing it to putrefy and rot in our colons causing gas, constipation, and bad digestion.

- We are by nature designed to eat fruits, vegetables, nuts and seeds.

Chapter 7 – Processed and refined foods

What is a processed food?

Processed foods are any type of food which has been altered by a process. That process can be cooking, freezing, canning, or drying. Not all processed foods are bad so here is how you can look out for the bad ones. Products such as "Oreos" are a great example of a bad processed food. They have high amounts of refined oils and are full of ingredients that many people can't pronounce, and you certainly wouldn't find in nature. On the other hand, you have something such as canned peaches which may have been heated during the canning process, and bathed in a sugary liquid, and have some natural preservatives added, such as Vitamin C or citric acid. Now you can see the contrast here, although of course a fresh peach would always be the healthiest option than a canned peach, but when in a pinch, it isn't a bad option either (especially if the other alternative is something such as Oreos). Also, there are frozen products which have simply been frozen on site, but this can be a very good thing because the manufacturer doesn't have to pick it unripe as it won't be travelling unripe. They can literally freeze it at optimum ripeness/nutrition/flavor, and send it directly to the store while keeping it frozen at all times. So although frozen vegetables or fruit may have undergone a process, it's not necessarily a bad one. Drying fruit and other products are another process, foods such as grapes are dried into raisins and can be a great way of storing them. They can also be added into cooking and are much more calorie dense making them great for snacking in combination with other dense naturally dry foods such as nuts and seeds. Cooking is a very common process that we use for many different reasons. It removes bacteria and germs from the food, breaks the food down so it's easier for our bodies to absorb. Usually it makes the food tastier too. Of course, you can have too much of a good thing and food can be overcooked and lose nutrients, and even burn which turns the food into carbon which can be harmful for us if eaten in big amounts. So not all processes are bad but some such as refining should be avoided in our foods.

What is a refined food?

Often people will get processed and refined foods mixed up. Refining a food item is a process in which the food is manipulated and often parts of it are taken away to achieve a totally different product. The process of refining oil from a sunflower seed where the seed is processed and only the oil is left, no other macronutrients such as carbohydrates or proteins, only fat. Oil is something we don't think about, we buy oil by the liter and are even told some oils such as "extra virgin olive oil" are healthy! Sugar is also another example of this, you take a crop such as sugar cane, juice it, and dry it out to form sugar crystals, what is left is almost pure carbohydrate, no fiber, and almost no nutrients. The most common refined products you will find are containing only one of each of the 3 macronutrients. Which can be sugar, or maltodextrin, which is a carbohydrate. Or protein powders, which are usually protein isolates from many different sources. Or oil, which is pure fat.

Why shouldn't I eat some refined foods?

It all boils down to what our body understands, so it can easily metabolize, assimilate and absorb the nutrients and fuel. Now let's compare 100g of peanuts; which contain on average: 567 calories, 49g of fat, 26g of protein and 16g of carbohydrate, most importantly 9g of fiber and many macronutrients. Compare that to peanut oil, which contains: 884 calories 100g fat, 0 protein and 0 carbohydrate, and almost no micronutrients. How do you think the body would respond to a peanut vs the refined peanut oil? The peanut would go into the body and the body would know how to efficiently use every macronutrient and micronutrient, and chances are wouldn't immediately be stored as fat. It would also be very filling and you would have to spend a lot of time chewing it, so the body would send the appropriate signals to tell you when to stop when you are full and satisfied. On the other hand, peanut oil would take maybe a few seconds to consume but take up much less volume in the stomach, despite being almost double the calories. The body would be sent into a state of shock and not know what had hit it. It would typically store most of it, if not all, of the oil as fat! Unless you were hugely active and the rest would try to be released through the pores, (usually as spots and grease on the skin). Have you ever eaten a lot of oily foods and then wondered why your face was greasy? So, as you could imagine this would not be great for weight loss. I'm not saying refined foods should be avoided 100%, but certainly refined fats should not be part of your daily diet.

What are some exceptions?

Refined sugar has a bad rep, mainly due to the fact it is often paired with fats, such as doughnuts, chocolate cake, etc, but it's not the sugar that's bad, it's the fats and possibly chemicals combined with the sugars. Carbs and refined sugars are guilty by association, which is why these same people who demonize refined sugar or even carbs can talk about how fruit (mostly sugar, water, vitamins and minerals) can be considered good. Refined sugar has never been proven to cause weight gain and has even been shown to reverse diabase and such with examples such as the Walter kempner rice diet where the people would just eat, white rice, sugar and juice. As a side effect these people would also lean out. I honestly believe in todays busy world it's so easy to not get in enough carbs which is so important for everything that we do and adding some refined sugar to your smoothie, oatmeal etc can be a great way to make sure you eat enough and are ready to tackle the day! A great example too would be for an athlete, they should definitely consume refined sugar, whether added to their water bottle or in the form of gels, it will fuel their workout, aid recovery and improve performance!

- Processed foods are any type of food that has been altered by a process.

- Not all processed foods are bad, as cooking and freezing are a type of process as well.

- Products such as Oreos are a great example of a bad processed food.

- A great example of a good processed food is a baked potato.

- Refined sugar can be great to add to supplement your fuel intake to make sure you get in enough calories or fuel during workouts.

- Refining removes some or most of the food's essential parts. Such as removing fats, proteins, or carbs, and isolating them to make products such as oil, protein powder, and sugar.

- Oil is 100% fat and sugar is 100% carbohydrates.

Chapter 8 – Whole foods and intuitive eating

What is a whole food?

A simple way of describing a whole food is a food item that is 100% natural made from the Earth; such as a potato. It has had little processing, and is free from artificial substances. So, a baked potato with some paprika and herbs added is still a whole food. On the contrary, a McDonald's hash brown comprises of Potato (91%), Canola Oil, Salt, Dextrose (from maize), Emulsifier (471), Preservative (450, 222), Antioxidant (330), Natural Pepper Extracts. NOT a whole food. You can see the difference. So if you cook or blend the food such as baking a potato or blending a smoothie it's still a whole food, but has undergone a process of cooking to be edible. Orange juice from juicing an orange however is not a whole food as it leaves behind much of the proteins and fiber contained in the orange, so our body will interpret it very differently. Which can trigger a blood sugar spike due to the lack of fiber, (more on this next).

Why whole foods?

Foods that are in their natural and whole state, which contain all the macronutrients and micronutrients that nature designed are perfect for human consumption. From a weight loss perspective eating 1kg of apples which contain all the natural macro and micro nutrients such as fiber and protein. The fiber actually helps slow our blood sugar spike down which keeps us in a fat burning state. Having your blood sugar high or consuming foods that make it high such as fruit juices, sugar, and fats, cause us to be in a fat storing mode, again not good for fat loss. Even consuming the refined sugar with some fiber such as berries has even been shown to have a lowering effect on the blood sugar spikes.

Whole foods are less calories but more volume

Typically, whole foods have much greater volume and are more filling than their refined counterparts. For example; eating 1kg of grapes vs drinking 1kg of grape juice. Or eating 1kg of sugar canes vs eating 1kg of sugar. Not to mention the difference in calories. 1kg of grapes might be around 500 calories vs 1kg of grape juice around 1000 calories, which is double the calories, and yet you can consume much, much more grape juice. It's very easy to overeat with more refined foods and typically you will find them much more calorie dense.

Intuitive eating

Have you ever seen an animal such as a rabbit or horse? They have fields of greens and grass in front of them, but yet they are still able to stop when they are full? Have you ever eaten too many packets of cookies or cakes and then suddenly felt almost sick? Well this will be because you have overeaten. Do you think the same would be possible with fruit, rice, potatoes, broccoli and beans? When I sit down to a meal of whole foods, before I feel very full in my stomach I become less interested in the food and suddenly those baked potatoes don't seem as appetizing to me, and the thought of them almost repulses me. On the other hand, I wouldn't naturally know when to stop with store bought cookies (mainly due to the excess fats). Have you ever seen an animal weigh their meals on a scale? Or count the calories they ate that day? I'm sure you haven't, maybe this made you chuckle. Now I'm not going to say DON'T weigh your food items as it often has a purpose. For example, when you're making a recipe or using dried products which swell considerably such as oats or beans. Eventually you will know exactly what the right portion for you is, and you will be able to eat until satiation and stop. Don't be afraid of leaving some on your plate. That can be stored in the fridge or freezer for another day, and the next time you can cook less. I would advise for people who are new to this to not have any distractions in the background, such as TV or a mobile phone, as these things can keep us distracted and stop us from listening to our body's natural signals. In time though, you will adapt.

Why eat like this?

If you ate 200 calories too much for your body, for every meal, 3 meals a day, over a week, could you imagine how that can add up? Now I'm not saying your body will automatically store all or even any of this excess as fat, but it CERTAINLY WILL NOT help any efforts of weight loss. Now if you sat and paid attention to your food, and stopped when you fell fully satisfied, (not when you've finished your plate), you will most naturally eat the right number of calories that you need for your body.

Calorie counting... should you do it?

As I said above, animals in nature don't weight their food out before each meal. But then again animals don't deal with dried products which can swell up much more than double their original form. I would advise keeping an eye on your calorie consumption when beginning any new lifestyle. To make sure you're eating enough, as when you are cutting out all of the junk such as meat, dairy and processed products, you will find that plant foods are a lot less calorie dense. This isn't a bad thing because you can eat much, much more to the point where if you're in a restaurant people may give your piled high plates a very strange glance. Usually people will have a small amount of meat with very small amount of starches and vegetables. You are no doubt familiar with the 2000 calories a day for women, and 2500 calories a day for men, (depending on which country you are from). This is a very generic figure not taking into account things like muscle mass and activity levels. How many calories do you need? That depends on YOU. If you are female, and eating 3000 calories a day, feel great, exercise plenty, are maintaining weight, and don't get excessively hot, or have bad period cycles then carry on. However, if you are a female, eating 3000 calories a day, gaining weight like crazy without a restrictive past, sedentary, and have awfully heavy periods and feel bloated after each meal, then for sure listen to these signs and decrease your calories and portions. On the contrary, you could be eating 1500 calories, losing weight rapidly but not have much energy, feel lethargic all the time, and not able to hit your workouts properly, and feel super hungry when you finish a meal, then increase your calories and portions.

Overtime with intuitive eating and eating the right foods you will be able to judge how much exactly your body needs, of course some days will vary. Once you have an understanding on how much you need to eat and when you feel full, I'd challenge you to stop counting calories and just eat until satiation!

Don't rely 100% on wholefoods

Everything I said about wholefoods I stand by, but to be realistic, we don't live as nature intended, so why should we eat the diet it intended for us? We are busy, too little time to cook up potatoes and veg or to sit down and eat a huge volume of food to get in the calories. Some of us like to ride our bikes for hours on end or are running around doing errands whilst looking after troublesome children. On busy days, feel free to eat some clean refined carbohydrate foods like white rice, refined sugar, pasta, pizza etc. On the bike or during exercise, feel free to add sugar to your water bottle during the rides. But to make your diet nutritious as possible, try to stick to as much wholefoods as possible and supplement with refined sugar, white rice, pasta etc...

My experience eating mostly wholefoods

Around late 2016 I implemented an almost all wholefoods diet on myself, continued my very active lifestyle, continued cycling etc. I continued not fueling during rides unless it was using only dried fruits such as raisins. I found overtime I was in a severe calorie deficit, because whilst I still packed in all the food I wanted, I could only eat around 4000 calories a day on average, despite burning 5000-7000 calories some days. This later on caused my metabolism to crash and I gained weight to the point where it was almost unreal. As I write this, I'm 98kg, the past really does come back to haunt you. I definitely DON'T recommend a purely wholefoods diet if your living an active lifestyle and actually exercising etc. Feel free to take refined sugars on rides, eat big portions of pasta or white rice on big ride days etc if you want to avoid getting post starvation obesity. But ofc, eat plenty wholefoods and use the refined as a supplement.

Chapter 8 Conclusion

- Whole foods are foods that are in their whole and natural state, such as baked potatoes as opposed to potato chips.

- Whole foods contain fiber, which helps keep us fuller for longer, and also helps reduce the insulin spike from fatty foods.

- Whole foods are intact and contain all the natural micronutrients. Carbohydrates, proteins, and fats.

- Whole foods are less calories, but more volume when compared to refined foods. Leaving you more satiated, without a chance of overeating.

- You can ditch calorie counting and start intuitive eating, just eat as much whole foods as you desire, and your body will tell you to stop when your body is full.

- We can't be purists though and rely 100% on wholefoods, sometimes with active lifestyles we have to supplement with some refined sugars, starches etc.

Chapter 9 – Sauces, condiments and salt

Should you avoid salt?

There is no easy yes or no answer to this. Salt can be a good thing for you, allow you to enjoy your meals and make them tastier. However, salt can also cause you to gain water weight if eaten too much, as mentioned in <u>Chapter 2</u>. Depending on how much salt you consume, and your activity levels, and the environment you live, salt can be harmful or harmless. As advised in <u>Chapter 7</u> try to stay away from processed foods as they can be very high in salt and much worse chemicals. If you are in a hot country and exercise a lot, you may not even need to worry about your salt consumption as you could sweat it out daily. But if you are in a colder climate and sedentary, or not doing much exercise, it can definitely make a difference. Some people have different reasons to add or take away salt. Personally, I add a bit of salt to my evening meal, so I don't have to go to the toilet several times during the night, which disturbs my sleep. I've found no other ill effects from it though as I'm very active. Another theory behind avoiding salt is that the fat cells are actually where the body stores water weight. So if you have a lot of water weight that the body needs to store, the body may be less eager to remove the fat, thus making it harder to lose weight.

How much salt is too much?

Again, there is no correct answer here, as I've mentioned it is depended on several variables. But I'd give as a guideline a figure of about 1000mg or no more than 1g of salt per day. But if you're sweating a lot and live a very active lifestyle, no doubt you'll want more, if you feel light headed, that's usually an indicator of lack of salt, so be sure to add in salt that day. Don't limit salt if you're an athlete or someone cycling or running for more than 1 hour daily or 7+ hours a week.

Are condiments ok?

When I spoke about wholefoods back in Chapter 8 and trying to eat foods as natural and whole as possible, I didn't mention about how to have them or flavor them. I'm not going to tell anyone to have their foods plain as that's not going to be sustainable for life, and no doubt people will become very miserable. So, I will say add a small amount of soy sauce or hot chili sauce, (or whatever sauce that you appreciate), to your meals. But don't drown it in sauce, so you can still appreciate the subtle flavors of whole foods, and allow your taste buds to change to learn to love the taste of natural foods. A word of caution though, try to get a sauce with the least ingredient. For example, many sauces can have weird chemical ingredients like; Monosodium glutamate, (also known as MSG), so be sure to avoid that like the plague! Tabasco sauce is a great example of a very minimal ingredients sauce, with just a few simple ingredients (peppers, vinegar and salt). As for making your own sauces using natural spices such as cumin, coriander and turmeric, go right ahead. I often make the most delicious curry's using mainly these simple and nutrient rich spices!

Making your own sauces

Many of you will be accustomed to buying premade sauces but have you ever stopped to consider making your own healthy alternatives? A homemade sauce could be equally as tasty, (if not tastier), with minimal and healthier ingredients. There are literally endless supplies of recipes online for sauces, which you can customize your own tastes as well. Something you can do is make a batch of a sauce, for example you could make a lentil curry at the beginning of the week and have it with many different dishes over the week as a sauce to give it delicious flavor.

Chapter 9 Conclusion

- Salt in small doses can be ok.

- If you're an athlete or very active, DON'T limit salt

- If you have to eat salty foods, try to add salt yourself, or eat the least processed salty foods.

- Experiment and see how salt works for your body.

- Excess salt can reduce weight loss, if you are struggling to lose weight but doing everything else right, then look into your salt intake and reduce if necessary.

Chapter 10 – Intermittent fasting for weight loss?

What is intermittent fasting?

Setting you're eating windows to be typically as short as possible such as 1 hour or 8 hours a day which is very common. Typically, it involves skipping breakfast, which has always been instilled in us since birth, "breakfast is the most important meal of the day" and in my opinion it really is. Breaking that fast is very important to rev up your metabolism and get your brain and body functioning correctly with plenty of fuel. Scientists and dietitians and people have come up with this theory to mimic nature, the fact we wouldn't have necessarily eaten all day, based on the assumption we ate a lot of meat. This is NOT the case, we are frugivores and we would have relied on many of our calories from tree ripened, super sweet fruits. Also, we'd have eaten and cooked starchy tubers such as potatoes, sweet potatoes etc. Living in a jungle with fruit trees everywhere, we would have had no need to go hungry, even just eating an apple from a tree as a quick snack while we're gathering fire wood or foraging would have broken a fast. We would of eaten when hungry, stopped when full and I'm sure of gathered food for the next meal or several meals too. Many people have taken intermittent fasting to extreme and practice OMAD or one meal a day and report benefits, but they seem to be short lived, many of these people were even thriving on a vegan diet before doing this and quickly dropped off. The fact of the matter is, we're not carnivores and therefore we are more grazers, we simply can't fit our daily caloric requirements into one meal, our stomachs won't allow it, especially on whole foods only. Now of course there would have been times, we skipped eating due to some unforeseen circumstance, but we certainly wouldn't have looked at clocks and not eaten for another 2 hours etc.

My experience intermittent fasting

Intermittent fasting can and no doubt will help you lose weight in the short term, excessive fasted cardio in combination with intermittent fasting quickly lost me 140lbs. But in the long term, it will mess up your adrenals and thyroid and cause weight gain. As I write this, I'm currently 98kg, 20kg heavier than I was! This is all due to me having a past of intermittent fasting and relying heavily on wholefoods despite doing plenty of cardio and creating a huge calorie deficit. For a while now, ever since hearing about intermittent fasting messing up your adrenals, I've been trying to eat as often as possible, often eating every 2-4 hours or so, never letting myself go starving. I definitely in the past experienced some signs of adrenals fatigue such as insomnia and waking up randomly in the nights etc. also some days feeling fatigued. That seems to be fixed now for me since eating plenty of times a day.

So how often or how many meals should I eat?

The typical 3 meals with the addition of some snacks on occasion works very well for me, but maybe you'd prefer 6 smaller meals or 2 big meals and snacks. I would just say to start with the typical 3 meals a day and if you feel like a snack in-between have it! If you feel like eating 2 big meals a day, just make sure your having a few snacks in-between to keep your blood sugar up and stop any moodiness or bonking during exercise.

The different types of intermittent fasting

There are a few types of intermittent fasting, one of the most popular ones is the 16/8 method where you eat during an 8-hour period leaving 16 hours fasted. Another is the 5:2 method where 2 days a week you eat minimal calories (around 500), this one I've also tried, and it was horrible! I got literally no results from it. It was not sustainable at all in my opinion. Then there is the eat-stop-eat method, where you don't eat anything from dinner one day until dinner the next day. I've never tried this one, but it sounds horrible too...

Chapter 10 Conclusion

- Intermittent fasting is unnatural for humans and only in rare or extreme cases would we have practiced this in nature

- Intermittent fasting means: Eating only during a certain time frame each day, usually a small window, such as 8 hours.

- Keeping eating regularly will keep your metabolism high and keep your blood sugar up so you think clearly and be your best self!

- I DON'T recommend intermittent fasting as it will stress out your hormones, lower your insulin sensitivity and set you up for weight gain in the future!

Chapter 11 – Calories and adaptive thermogenesis

Calories in, calories out right?

There's so much basic info out there about calories, people honestly thinking, a calorie is a calorie and if I eat X number of calories I will lose, maintain or gain, I call serious bullshit on this approach! As I mentioned in Chapter 8 animals don't count calories and we wouldn't have dreamed about it initially, we would of eaten until satisfied and stopped when we were full. We wouldn't have had access to such fatty, junky foods, with only nuts and seeds, it would have been a pain in the ass to deal with, not coming prepackaged and deshelled as they do today. And ofc oils weren't a thing, this is the real reason people need to calorie count, they are eating a SAD diet with most of their calories coming from fat and protein, bulking foods. The same way a cow can eat grass all day and stay healthy weight, yet if the farmer feeds them soy which is a fatty legume their weight skyrockets. So, if you're eating the proper human fuel which is carbohydrates, there's literally no need to count calories, your body will let you know when your full. Here's a perfect example of this, I usually ride with 100g of sugar per hour on my bike and when I get home, I eat fruit for breakfast or sometimes if it was a hectic training morning, I'll have another liter of sugar and lemon water beforehand. When I come to eat the fruit, I find myself eating around half as much as I used to eat before I implemented sugar during the rides, despite sugar not having any fiber and such, the body still recognizes the calories, and therefore tells me to stop eating, as I've already had enough carbs. When I say carbohydrates, I mean the clean ones, like rice, fruit, pasta, corn, grains, sugar etc. NOT doughnuts, takeaway pizzas, candies, chocolate bars, as they are usually half or more calories coming from fat, most of which will get stored, assuming you're not exercising a lot. Another thing to note here is it's really hard for the body to store carbohydrates as fat contrary to popular belief, the body will usually store excess carbohydrates in the muscles as glycogen first, then it will begin to remove sugars in the form of urine making for some sweet pee! If that fails, your body will heat you up, using a process known as dietary thermogenesis, so if you've eaten too much, your pee may smell sweeter and you may have a bead of sweat on your forehead, or find yourself removing items of clothes. Typically, the body will only store carbs as fat during post starvation obesity and this is an extreme survival mechanism. So as long as your eating the right diet which should be rich in carbohydrates, low in fat and protein with around 80+% of calories coming from carbohydrates which if you eat fruit, grains, potatoes, refined sugars you will easily be eating 90%, there's no need to count.

My weight gain due to adaptive thermogenesis story

I always thought "metabolic damage" or adaptive thermogenesis was a myth, something that recovering anorexics got, or something that would never concern me, how wrong was I!

After getting SUPER close to my goal weight within about 7kg at the time (based on estimated lean body mass) I began to rapidly gain weight. At the time I thought, maybe it's because I was exercising less, or maybe I'm eating TOO MUCH? The first time this happened was mid-late 2017 and I figured at the time, I was eating some fats and not exercising as much, so I ofc blamed that, as soon as I was back on the bike often, the weight cleared. Then come 2018 I was doing Deliveroo, somedays 12-hour sessions, eating predominantly wholefoods and taking potatoes, apples and some dried fruits with me as "fuel". Fast forward to October, I quit Deliveroo due to bad weather and dark evenings (which I would do most days) and for safety I took up a basic warehouse job over Christmas. During Christmas, I ate plenty of "treats" and had plenty of rest, ofc the weight piled on again and by 2019 I was around 5kg over my lowest weight. I started up Deliveroo again for the summer of 2019 as I figured the risks and the freedom was worth the potential risks and much better than some dead end, soul sucking job. Ofc the weight came off again despite not really eating much more (which was a BIG mistake), and I was 78kg. I stopped working Deliveroo in September

2019 due to moving to Spain, once we got to Spain, I resumed teaching English online and mainly used my bike for transport. My wife said I was looking "bigger" again and I weighed in and within 2 months I'd gained 12kg, which was blamed on some hummus sandwiches I'd made while visiting Spain and by "overeating" on carbs, something I'd always found impossible to do and always been told this and honestly believed it and still do! I figured though, I would have to "restrict" my calories, so I went down to 2500, I got really, really hungry during this phase, would be thinking about food 24/7, feeling unsatisfied during meals, despite trying to add in vegetables and such to try and bulk out the meal, ofc my body knew that vegetables weren't fuel.

 I actually maintained my weight during this and the thought of having to go lower to lose made me so sad. So I just kind of continued maintaining and my calories snook up as I'd stopped tracking, as I got sick of it, once we got to Thailand, I was like, I'm going to ride this weight off and began trying to do that, meanwhile weight staying the exactly the same? It wasn't too much longer, maybe 2 weeks in I had an accident on my way down the local Mountain (Doi Suthep) and I was left with a huge chunk missing out of my arm and due to my bike being broken, I wasn't able to ride for a good few weeks or so while it got repaired. I took some time for myself during the recovery and I'm not sure whether I saw an article or somebodies video, but It was just like one of those "ahah" moments and I realised that I had ALL of the same symptoms of somebody recovering from anorexia or another kind of eating disorder. I realised the thinking about food constantly, the huge appetite and hunger for food, planning "binges " on set days each week etc, was all signs that I wasn't getting in enough fuel for my bodies requirements, not to mention the post starvation obesity symptoms I experienced, despite not getting obese.

 It was at this point, I realised I needed to "go all in" and just eat to my hunger and eat as much as I wanted, which I've been doing since around March 2020 and so far I've gained about 10kg, but it seems to of calmed down now, in the first 2 weeks I was gaining almost 1lb of FAT a day! My appetite has calmed down a bit, there's some days when I have a big hunger and other days it feels more normal. I've implemented some light exercise in and am cycling about 6 hours a week + 3 hours strength at gym and I was up until this point doing 2 hours running, but it's became too painful with my weight, so I've stopped, I'll fill that with 2 hours cycling, averaging between 7-9 hours. I'm currently at 98kg as I write this and I've weighed this for over a week now, so I'm hoping the weight has plateaued and the only way is down. During this time, I've found myself watching Durianrider's videos to reprogram myself and get back on track, I'd fell for the orthorexic diets such as Dr gregor's and the SOS and whole foods movement and I now have less health than when I started which is ironic really. When I started this lifestyle, I ate all the carbs I could, rode my bike and lost weight. When I changed that formula, by not eating all the carbs I wanted, eating only whole foods and generally being too pure, I created a serious calorie deficit which really messed up my metabolism!

Chapter 11 Conclusion

- Don't worry about calories, just make sure you're eating enough high carb foods without fat or oil.
- Despite sounding counterintuitive, not eating enough can make you fat, as your body will remember and slow the metabolism so that when you do eat a generous amount again, it will take it all and store as much as fat as possible, ready for the next famine.
- You don't have to suffer from an eating disorder to get post starvation obesity, anyone who has eaten in a calorie deficit for a while, whether by accident because busy at work, or just through exercising and not putting enough back in.
- For the athletes, training fueled if vital, as you can easily fall into a serious calorie deficit otherwise as it's hard for the body to eat so many calories, vs drinking them or consuming as refined products.

Chapter 12 – Exercise and its role in weight loss

Humans are supposed to be active by nature

Firstly, without even talking about the weight loss aspect of which exercising can have on the body, I should talk about how natural it is to actually *move* the body instead of sitting in traffic in a car, or sitting all day at the office. In nature we would have had to walk or run everywhere whether it be to the trees or bushes to gather fruit and vegetables or to the local water source. Now to gather food we walk maybe 5-10 meters out of our front door and sit in a car, push a pedal, and turn a wheel, and we arrive at the supermarket where we buy our groceries. We then push a cart around with all of the goods and proceed to load them into our car. Originally, we would have walked or ran to a food source, handpicked it which could have taken hours, then most likely walked back with some kind of container carrying all of the food items. You see how few calories we actually burn now just by vehicles and supermarkets existing? It's no wonder obesity is at an all-time high, I'm sure if everyone had to walk 5-10km to the local food takeaway vs calling them on the phone to deliver people would be less incline to do so. It reminds me of a scene from the Movie "Wall E", where humans had become such fat slobs, they were moving around on motorized vehicles that they basically lived on all day, it had everything they needed. Their bodies were fat, and very weak through lack of use. Sadly, this world is almost already there if we don't act fast!

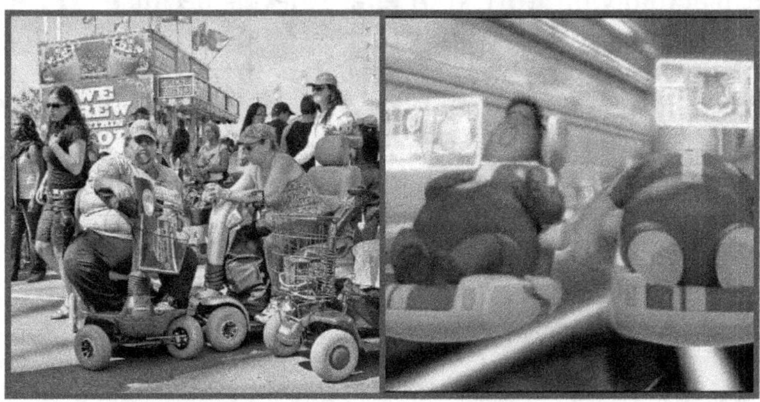

Why exercise?

The better question would be why not? I heard a saying which resonated with me a while back, and it went something like this; "Take care of your body, it's the only place you have to live." By exercising properly, you are definitely helping to prolong the body. What do you have to do with your day that is better than moving your body as we were intended to do like any animal does. For sure resting is good, but not all day.

First of all, exercise is great for burning excess fat calories each day to maintain, or help get you to a healthy weight. Exercise can be key in improving your mood by stimulating various brain chemicals which release "feel good" hormones. Regular exercise helps prevent or manage a wide range of health problems and concerns; including stroke, metabolic syndrome, type 2 diabetes, numerous of types of cancer, arthritis, and falls. It may sound counter intuitive but exercise can actually improve your energy levels because exercising forces the body to deliver more oxygen rich blood around the body which can help make you feel more awake. Exercise improves sleep by naturally aiding you to fall asleep faster, just don't exercise before bed or you may be too energized. Exercise can improve your life span and overall health by increasing your cardiovascular system which will allow your heart and lungs to be much more efficient at rest, giving you a lower resting heart rate, which is healthier!

When should you exercise?

You can exercise anytime during the day that suits you. I would not recommend exercising a few hours before bed though, as I said above it can leave you feeling energized. Personally, I prefer to exercise first thing in the morning to get it done with. That's also when I'm at my most motivated too. I would usually wake up, fill up my bottles with sugar or take some dates with me and exercise for 1-3 hours then come back home and have breakfast. Occasionally in the afternoon I would also exercise, sometimes to run errands on my bicycle, (I'll talk more about this later), and sometimes for fun. The best time to exercise is when it most suits your schedule, you're the most motivated at that time, and it'll be most sustainable for you, in which you can build into your lifestyle. (More on building a lifestyle later).

How does exercise affect weight loss?

When I first started my healthier eating back in May 2014, I was barely exercising and very sedentary, which really showed on my weight loss. Which despite being around the 300lb mark was nonexistent! I didn't lose any weight for well over 6 months which led me to do an extreme raw food only cleanse. Although I lost 10 or more pounds whilst doing this for a month, I felt tired and hungry all the time! It literally felt like I was fasting. As soon as I started consistent and real exercise in the form of cycling on May 2015, that's when I really started to see results. Exercising burns extra calories than your body does while at rest. Which in turn, (depending on how active you are), can create a calorie deficit. Which your body will have to find fuel from excess carbohydrates in the form of glycogen and fat, instead of food. Another thing that exercising does is damage muscles, so repair is needed whilst you're resting. So those extra calories will be used in the repairing of damaged bodily tissues. Both of these ramps up our metabolism which cause our BMR, (basil metabolic rate), to go up and thus the body burning more calories, (more on this in a later chapter). Too much exercise without adequate calories at a low body fat percentage on the other hand can cause the body to gain weight as it's fighting for survival and holding onto any excess fat stores you may have.

Zone training and how to optimize exercise for fat loss!

Whilst you're exercising, your body uses two main sources of fuel. Glycogen, which is basically a form of glucose stored in the body's tissues for use whilst exercising, and fat, which is rather self-explanatory. Different types of exercising will trigger different kinds of fuel being burnt. For example, many people use the traditional "Zones" for training. There can be different calculation methods, but don't worry about that for now. The best way to calculate *your* zones, whether they come from heart rate data, or power data, is to do an FTHR or FTP test. Information on how to do it and then calculate it can be found on this here and here. Now that you've read those articles I can talk about the different zones and what they mean for fat loss. Zone 1 is a very easy zone where your will barely be out of breath, and you will burn mostly fat and a little bit of glycogen. Zone 2 you will burn more fat and more glycogen but still more fat than glycogen ratio. Zone 2 can be an all day, endurance pace. Zone 3 burns more fat than zone 2 but also burns an equal amount of glycogen making it unsustainable for long periods, making zone 2 more efficient for long term fat burning goals. Zone 4,5 burn 90-100% glycogen which will basically be just last night's dinner getting burnt vs fat loss. Of course, you will gain fitness at these zones though, which can be good for sprinting, and time trial efforts. See the chart below.

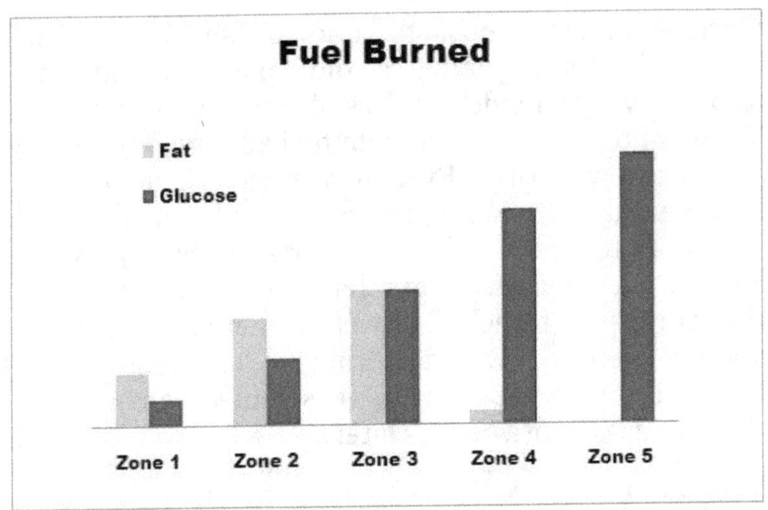

How much exercise should you do?

If you're just starting out, then by doing a few times a week you will no doubt massively increase your exercise anyway, so take things easy. Increasing exercise too quickly, and/or too soon, can be a recipe for disaster. Making you feel so fatigued or even result in injury. The best method, at least in my experience, is to introduce exercise gradually and increase it as you get fitter and healthier. Once you find yourself doing 4-5 times a week, see how you get on and you can increase the total duration of each workout. As for total volume, that all depends on you. Some athletes will do 20-40 hours a week of exercise, but for the purposes of weight loss you don't need to do that much. I wouldn't recommend this though for wright loss, I've done this in the past and it created a serious calorie deficit with left me with some adaptive thermogenesis and post starvation obesity, as it left my body with a serious deficit, so ofc it panicked and went into "starvation mode". Unless of course you would like to, and can pack in enough fuel and are physically and mentally capable. Even an average of around 1 hour per day (6-7 hours per week) should make a vast difference to your weight loss efforts, especially if you are coming from a sedentary background. I also found that during "rest weeks", or weeks where I was sick and not exercise, I would continue to lose weight. I believe this was due to my increased metabolism from the exercise, (more on this later).

Training smart vs training hard

Some people will try to push their bodies too far beyond their current limits which can lead to fatigue and having to take extra time off, or even injury. I remember once pushing myself too hard and getting sick with the flu which cost me 1-2 weeks of training. If I'd have backed off earlier, I no doubt wouldn't have gotten sick which would have allowed me to get more training load in. Which is the key to long term success. If you set yourself realistic goals and listen to your body, you can achieve more total workload than if you ignore your body's signals, and set yourself unrealistic goals. You have to think about the bigger picture. Is this 1 session going to make you miss 5 more sessions? What's missing out on 10 minutes of zone 5 going to do vs missing out on 5 total sessions?

How to EASILY fit exercise into your daily life

A big reason or, in my opinion, an excuse of why people don't exercise, either at all or even enough is; time. They say, "I don't have time", or "I'm too busy with work and my family", or something similar. An easy way of getting rid of that excuse is exercising on the way to where you are going! Yes, you heard me right. If you're like most people, when you need an item from a nearby store you will drive or catch the bus 1-10km to retrieve this item, when you could walk or even cycle there. I know walking 10km often isn't practical for time but I'm sure everybody had time to walk 1-2km each day at least. Most people will work less than 10km from their house and yet they will sit in a car stuck in traffic for anything up to 2 hours just to get there. Or even worse on a stuffy bus or train. Why bother when you can breeze past all of the cars stuck in traffic on your bicycle? It's becoming a very popular way of commuting in big cities nowadays. As nobody in the right mind would want to be stuck in traffic for hours on end. Just imagine how much exercise you could achieve each week by simply switching to ride a bicycle, or walking to work each day! If everybody did this, think of how congestion free the roads would be and how clean the air would be to breath. Personally, I've been pretty much car free for years now. I have a rack and panier for my bicycle, and anything that needs carrying I either use that, or bring a backpack as well. I do "market hauls" and carry 20kg bunches of bananas on my back, 10kg of sweet potatoes on my bike rack, along with around 5kg of vegetables too for a whopping total of 35kg. Now I'm not saying you should do this to this extreme, but for sure if you want some light groceries, you should consider getting a bike with a basket, rack, panier, or just a sturdy and comfortable backpack to carry your shopping. There are so many ways you can sneak exercise into your daily life without even setting out to exercise directly. Since I have been focusing on calisthenics training to build muscle and tone up my body, I haven't really been on actual bike rides where I set out just to ride for a while now. But I still find myself using my bike for 5-10 hours a week, by just using it for my main transport. Now I'm not suggesting to get rid of your vehicle and never use it again. I'm simply offering many scenarios when you can easily switch being lazy and driving 1-2km, to riding your bike there instead. Vehicles of course have their place for long distances and for carrying very heavy goods. So even without setting out to directly exercise you can still get many hours of exercise in, which is good for your health and great for the planet!

Fasted Training for weight loss?

You've probably heard of people doing fasted training and recommending it for maximum fat loss, I even had this mindset, that if I ate before or during a ride, I'd just be burning that food and not the fat on the body. The opposite is true really, because doing fasted training will, overtime slow your metabolism and cause the body to be in starvation mode, during this time, yes it will b urn more fat, but it will also teach your body to prepare for the next famine and it will begin to hold onto it and you'll find your fat stores staying the same on the scales, or worse, as soon as the situation eases up, maybe you go on holiday or take a week off the bike, you're body will soak up all that fuel and turn it into fat. This also isn't mentioning the stress it does to your adrenal glands, which have to produce adrenaline to keep you fueled throughout the ride, which is not only toxic for you liver and can cause a sluggish liver down the line, but also tire your adrenal glands out, as they are only meant to be used in fight or flight situations. Always have a little fruit or fuel before a ride and during if practical. For rides under 1 hour, you can just have a piece of fruit, some gels or maybe a little smoothie. I'd recommend 100g of carbs/hour on anything over 1 hour though. Best way to do that is to add 100g sugar into your water bottle, you can also add some fruit juice such as lemon, lime or orange juice to give it a pleasant flavor and extra vitamins/minerals.

Cardio or strength training for fat loss?

There are two main types of exercise which can do many different things and are for people with different goals. Cardio which is usually running, cycling, swimming and activities which have a low impact on muscles but a high impact on the cardiovascular system, (heart and lungs). Cardio can be very effective for weight loss in the long and short term, as it directly burns fat stores from the body. So, you can see results almost immediately, even starting from as little as 20 or 30 minutes. In the long term you can increase the time you spend doing cardio due to your fitness improving, allowing you to burn even more fat. Another thing cardio training can do is increase your metabolism by forcing your body to burn extra calories and store carbohydrates as glycogen to replenish the muscles, also allowing you to eat more and have a bigger appetite. Cardio will also build small but lean style muscles. Think marathon runner vs 100m sprinter. In my opinion cardio should definitely be a large part of any weight loss program. Strength training usually involves much slower motions or reps as they are usually called in which the body pushes or pull a weight, whether it's their own body in the form of pushups, pull-ups or some other bodyweight exercise, or actual weights such as dumbbells or the weight machines. When the body is pushed to the limits, whether that's by doing a mixture of heavy weights and reps/sets, or just maximum reps until fatigue. When done correctly, your body repairs or replaces damaged muscle fibers through a cellular process where it fuses muscle fibers together to form new muscle protein strands or myofibrils. These repaired myofibrils increase in thickness and number, to create muscle hypertrophy (growth). Short term strength training burns very few calories as your heart rate doesn't usually get very high enough for it to increase your metabolism. Long term, the more muscle you gain, the more calories your body burns at rest to function correctly so when you start your weight loss journey. You should also incorporate some strength, although it won't make you look slim as quick as cardio, it will ramp up your metabolism and allow you to burn through more fat in a day. I would recommend a big focus on cardio to start with and some time spent strength training to increase your metabolism over time. Another thing to note is, if you just do cardio, when you do eventually slim down, you may end up looking too skinny or spindly. I certainly did. Had I have known about this; I would have incorporated strength training earlier too. Once you are towards the end of your weight loss, or in the toning phase, I would recommend focusing more on strength training and just maintaining your cardio a few times a week, and during commutes of course.

Chapter 12 Conclusion

- Remain as active as possible, as humans were originally. (DON'T let modern day customs make you lazy).

- Exercising is very healthy for the body and part of a healthy lifestyle.

- Find a balance between doing too much and too little exercise that works for you.

- Exercising ramps up your metabolism, making fat loss easier, even at rest.

- Use zone training, such as zone 1-3 to burn the most amount of fat possible

- Train smart and don't make training too hard.

- DON'T do fasted rides, always fuel before and or during the ride.

- Incorporate exercise into your daily lifestyle by making changes such as cycling or walking to work, instead of driving or catching the bus.

- Cardio is great for short term and long-term weight loss by directly burning fat from the body.

- Strength training is good for long term weight loss, as when you store more muscle your metabolism increases, burning more fat at rest.

Chapter 13 – The metabolism

What is the metabolism?

Metabolism is a term that is used to describe all chemical reactions involved in maintaining the living state of the cells and the organism. The speed of which your body uses calories (fuel), to complete these tasks can vary depending on many factors. For example, if you are a young, sedentary, short and petite female then your calorie expenditure each day would be small. However, if you're a young, active, tall and muscular female then your calorie expenditure will be much, much higher.

Slow metabolism vs fast metabolism

With a slow metabolism; you will typically burn less calories each day and usually your appetite will be less to meet that. Overeating could cause some weight gain and you might find that you gain weight easier than others. Or you may have trouble losing weight, feel tired all the time, have a difficult time staying warm, experience hair loss, and if you're a female, even period loss. This is because due to your lifestyle or lack of food intake, your body has had to slow down or shut off completely, many natural processes. You will also experience things such as slower digestion and inability to concentrate. This is a natural survival process that humans and animals have. For example, hair isn't needed on the body for you to stay alive, so naturally your body will stop this process (resulting in hair loss). Your body will divert resources to major organs and the brain to continue living. As for a fast metabolism; you will experience increased weight loss, increased body heat, more bowel movements, increased energy, and often the inability to sit still. Neither extreme is good and can be medically diagnosed as hypothyroidism which is; essentially too little thyroid hormones, causing our bodies to function too slowly or in simple terms (slow metabolism). Or hyperthyroidism which is the opposite; too many thyroid hormones increasing our metabolism too much for our bodies (fast metabolism).

Can the metabolism be increased?

Don't be fooled into thinking that you need to be a certain height, or age to have a high metabolism. The metabolism can be naturally and healthy speed up or even slowed down by actions you take. For example, being sedentary and not eating much food will automatically slow down your metabolism, whereas being active and eating plenty of food will speed it up.

So high metabolism equals weight loss?

Pretty much yes. Unless of course you are eating so much, or doing so little exercise, that you offset this. It's all about increasing your metabolism naturally and sustainably, which can allow you to burn more calories throughout the day.

How to increase metabolism for weight loss?

Exercising, eating whole foods and remaining active will over time speed up your metabolism as there will naturally be more going off for your body to fuel each day. Simply cycling to work and even in a sedentary job, getting up often to move or fidgeting on a fit ball can increase your metabolism and make you burn more calories at rest.

Basil metabolic rate (BMR)

Your BMR is the number of calories each day you will burn at rest. Following the above tips, whether it's gaining muscle, keeping active and eating good whole foods, (which use more calories to burn than refined foods), will increase your BMR. The healing process of damaged muscle tissue and improving your fitness will increase your BMR naturally.

Calorie restriction and slow metabolism

Restricting calories or your food intake and having a slow metabolism go hand in hand. Starving your body will make your body slow down it's processes as it's not getting enough fuel, this in turn as I mentioned can cause the whole host of negative effects that I mentioned earlier. This in turn will have a negative effect on weight loss in the long term, so this is not a good approach for anyone considering losing weight.

Chapter 13 Conclusion

- Metabolism is a term that is used to describe all the chemical reactions involved in maintaining the living state of the cells and the organism.

- Slow metabolism burns less calories at rest, resulting in negative side effects such as weight gain, natural bodily processes being shut down such as hair growth, the reproductive system, and lowering the human growth hormone, resulting in less muscle growth.

- Fast metabolism can result in excess weight loss, excess heat, hunger, and also cause the human growth hormone to grow, resulting in bigger muscular gains

- The metabolism can be increased by being active and eating enough fuel for your body's needs.

- BMR is the number of calories your body burns at rest to keep you alive.

Chapter 14 – Forming a lifestyle

As I spoke about in <u>Chapter 3</u> and the following chapters, fad diets and "get slim quick" schemes, don't work long term. So, you may be thinking, how do I turn all of this information you have given me into a lifestyle? To start, you don't do anything too extreme. For example, if you are sedentary and eating 1500 calories of junk food each day, then go to, cycling 4 hours and eating 5000 calories each day, would be a ridiculous transition to make within a few day or week period. On the other hand, if you decided to stop counting calories but ate as many healthy calories as your appetite required, whilst cycling slowly to work and back for 1 hour total a day (30 minutes each way), you could see how that could be a much more sustainable difference to implement over a few days or weeks. Starting off, you might not be able to make it all the way to work on the bike, so maybe you could cycle for 15 minutes around the block to build up.

Swapping out healthy food for unhealthy

Also finding and eating food that you actually enjoy is important. For example, maybe your go-to meal was a Spaghetti Bolognese with all of that greasy ground beef, added olive oil, and cheese slathered on top of refined white spaghetti. We could substitute that unhealthy ground beef for lentils, take out the oil and have a delicious and healthy lentil Bolognese on top of whole grain pasta with nutritional yeast for cheesiness on top. You don't have to go without the foods you enjoy. But rather adapt and make the healthy swaps, from the "bad foods", to the "good, natural, whole foods". Raw foodists have been doing this since they started, instead of just eating fruit and greens in their plain and natural state, they would often make smoothies, decadent desserts with soaked nuts and seeds, and make sauces for their salads all to make and replace their go-to cooked meals they ate before they are fully raw. There are so many healthy ways of enjoying the food you love. A great example of this is with ice cream. Did you know that you can freeze bananas, then put them into your blender or food processor with some berries, powders, or other flavorings to make different flavor "nice creams"? So you're eating healthy fruit, getting in vital nutrients, and yet you're satisfying your cravings for unhealthy junk food like as Ben and Jerry's Ice cream.

Getting into the active vs sedentary mindset

Have you ever taken an elevator up 2 or even 4 flights of stairs? Are you the kind of person who takes the escalator and just stands still vs walking up the stairs? Do you drive 1-5km to work or to the grocery store? If you answered yes to any of these questions, then you can definitely work on changing your mindset and habits to a more active way of life. It's as easy as walking up the stairs for a few flights instead of taking the lift, or cycling 5km to work instead of driving your car. Now of course if you need to go up 20 flights of stairs, or go 100km to work each day. I'm not suggesting you walk or cycle all of that, unless you want to challenge yourself! But you get what I'm saying about how easily you can become more active if you just allow yourself to get into the mindset.

Being healthy should be a lifestyle

Being healthy, exercising well and eating healthy for a few weeks or just a month won't really get you anywhere in the long run. As you'll just go back to your unhealthy ways. Who knows, maybe you will gain back more weight than you started, which is more common than you would think due the metabolism being slowed as I've mentioned before. It's the same with exercise, if you just do it once or for a few weeks then stop, you will lose all of the good benefits that you have gained. So vow to start a healthy lifestyle that will be with you for the rest of your life, you owe it to yourself and your body to start taking care of it in the form of good nutrition and exercise. Ask yourself this: can I eat this way for the rest of my life without feeling restricted or miserable? Can I sustain this amount of exercise for the rest of my life without feeling too fatigued, or not having time for anything else? If you answered NO to both or one, then you need to adjust your lifestyle to make it sustainable. For example, if you have tried 3 hours exercise per day but found it unsustainable due to fatigue or other commitments.

Maybe you can only get out twice a week for 3 hours but you could manage to get out 4 times a week for 2 hours, (which would be more workload). Do you see where I am going with this? It's the same with food. You need to make it sustainable so that you enjoy it and can eat this way indefinitely. I'm not saying every week has to be the same, for sure some weeks you will have a "treat" meal, or have a day off exercise because life got in the way or you didn't feel motivated, you're only human after all.

Design your lifestyle to suit you

So, let's say you have a "9-5 job". You normally leave the house at 8am, drive 10km in traffic to your job and arrive there around 8:55am, giving you just enough time to clock in and take off your coat. If this is the case, you can quite possibly set off at 8am and cycle to work and arrive for 8:30-8:45 (quite easily), giving you enough time to freshen up, clock in and take off your coat. So a simple change like that could be made and that would give you 60-90 minutes cycling each day 5 days a week (300-450 minutes or 5-7.5 hours). What if it's raining that day or you are running late or your bike needs a service? Be prepared, as with any lifestyle modification you will need to prepare. Cars are usually low maintenance in 2017, but bikes are still very simple in comparison and need more maintenance. So be sure to plan ahead. Keep your bike well maintained. As with anything, look after it and it will look after you. As for rain, it's very possible to go out with the correct clothing attire and fenders and not get too dirty. On the other hand, it can be slippery in the rain so really the choice is yours to access the situations and if you deem it unsafe due to pouring rain then so be it. It won't rain every day though, I'm sure, and if it does, consider relocating! As for eating, maybe you're work has a canteen but the food is bad. In that case, be sure to prepare food the night before to take along with you. You can even cook extra the night before and have leftovers as the next day's lunch. Meal prepping can be a very useful way of staying organized for these such times and allow you to not have to eat bad food. For everyone it will be different, some people will struggle with fitting in exercise, some people will struggle with preparing meals. There are always ways to overcome these things, whether it's commuting to work via bicycle and cycling on the weekend, or preparing a big batch of meals on the Sunday and freezing them, the only thing getting in the way is your excuses, (more on this on the next chapter).

Getting to bed early enough

Another thing I'd love to mention is that getting the right amount and quality of sleep each night is not only ideal for weight loss but it's almost a prerequisite. If you aren't getting enough sleep then your hormones can be out of balance and out of balance hormones can be a recipe for weight gain, not weight loss! You only need to see a girl who has gone on the contraceptive pill, (which is basically hormones in a pill), often they can gain weight, get acne, all of these things are controlled by hormones. So go to bed early and be early to rise if possible, but make sure you wake up feeling well rested every morning, ideally you will even wake before your alarm, not to it.

Stay hydrated

Many people underestimate the power of remaining hydrated. Often people will feel tired mid-afternoon and reach for the coffee and snacks, but it's often dehydration that is causing this. Ideally you should be peeing relatively clear, almost white wine colored, not apple juice colored, or yellow. Yellow pee can be a sign of dehydration and it's not great for digestion, and weight loss. Also keeping hydrated will keep you feeling fuller, sometimes we can mistake thirst for hunger and go for the bad foods.

Chapter 14 Conclusion

- Make changes that are sustainable for life!

- Swap out the unhealthy food for the healthy food, and continue to enjoy the same foods, but made healthy.

- Get into the active vs sedentary mindset. Take the stairs, NOT the elevator when possible.

- Get to bed early and get plenty of sleep.

- Stay hydrated, ideally peeing clear, or white wine colored, for optimal health and weight loss.

Chapter 15 – Excuses and what to do with them

Why we make excuses

Many people make excuses for many things in their life. For example, arriving to work late, they will tell their boss the reason was they were stuck in traffic, but the real reason was they didn't allow enough time and set off early enough, or they miscalculated the amount of time it would take to drive in the current traffic. Another excuse I see and hear far too often is "I don't have time to exercise" as I mentioned in the above chapters. There is always a way around this and it's mainly about being prepared. Making excuses like this makes us feel better and it often shifts blame either to other people or inanimate objects, therefore lifting the blame from us. Which often helps people feel better about themselves. The way we see ourselves after shifting the blame is in a much nicer light than if we accepted the reality of the truth. I was late because I snoozed my alarm and couldn't be bothered to get up. Or I didn't prepare my lunch last night, so I had to prepare it this morning. I should know about these things, I used to be the king of excuses. I always had an excuse for everything, the fact I often arrived at work at 7:02am when I should have been there at 7am. It was always the traffic's fault, not mine, for not leaving 5 minutes earlier. Why I was so fat... it was my genes that made me fat, not my lifestyle or my slow metabolism, not the fact I sat around like a slob most of the day and didn't exercise. You get the point I'm trying to make here anyway...

What should we do about it?

There will always be readily available excuses on hand to give you a security blanket from any given situation, but you need to learn to accept reality for what it is. So how should you handle situations without giving excuses? In my opinion the best option is prevention. Prevent possible scenarios where excuses might have to crop up. For example, using my "no nonsense approach" I could have a conversation with an excuse maker. The conversation could go a little like this:

I hear you were late for work today?

"Yes, the traffic was bad."

Couldn't you have left earlier for work?

"No, I didn't have time this morning."

Why don't you get up earlier?

"I am too tired to go to get up earlier"

Then why don't you go to bed earlier?

"I was watching TV"

Don't watch TV too late.

You see that I could almost argue indefinitely with this

excuse maker, it would be almost impossible to have a real conversation with them. Until eventually I trip them up from their own excuses. What can we learn from that conversation? Try to find solutions to problems rather than causing them, and then trying to cover them up with excuses. For example, this person could have said

"Yes, now I'm making excuses. Tomorrow I will go to bed earlier, which will allow me to wake earlier and I will leave earlier for work. This will allow me to get to work on time."

This was all caused by watching TV and going to bed late. Had this person not of gone to bed late, they could have woken earlier and not been in this mess. Each action has consequences and often one small action can have a snowball effect and the future consequences can become even larger. Really with these things, prevention is better than cure. No one is perfect and we all make mistakes, it's better to accept responsibility for them, learn from it and try not to make the same mistake again.

Lose your excuses and you'll find your results

So many people go through life using excuses for everyday things. Excuses will only hold you back from reaching your true potential. Whether it's with weight loss, fitness, or anything else in life. I used to make excuses a lot, and they only held me back. I woke up this morning knowing full well I should train calisthenics for 1 hour and then have a training ride with one of my clients, however it was raining. I could have woken up, cancelled calisthenics and the easy morning ride with my client, but what kind of message would that of sent out? I try to teach all of my clients a "no excuse mentality" and this would have taught the absolute opposite. On the other hand, had we of been training at serious speed, or in the mountains, it wouldn't have been an excuse to cancel due to pouring rain, but a safety issue. When I first started cycling, I could barely cycle 2km and when I did, I almost had an asthma attack, I could have quite easily used this as an excuse, sold my bike and gone back to my old ways. But I knew this would hold me back from achieving the weight loss I did today. It's only when I got out most mornings, trained hard, and ate the right foods, that I started seeing real results. So, the next time you want to be lazy and get out of exercising or eating right, ask yourself: Is this an excuse or a real reason? Can I really justify this excuse? Am I just saying this to try and clear my conscious? Will this excuse stop me from achieving the results I so badly want?

Chapter 15 Conclusion

- People make excuses to make themselves feel better about their failures.

- Try to prevent situations where you would need to make an excuse, or alternatively learn from these situations so they don't happen again.

- Stop making excuses, as they are only holding you back from achieving your full potential.

- Lose your excuses and you'll find your results!

Chapter 16 – Consistency is key

Results don't happen overnight

If you're like most people, then you're impatient and expect results overnight. You'll do a workout for a couple of days or even 1 day and expect to see either weight loss or muscle gains immediately. Sorry to dishearten you, but these things don't happen overnight and don't listen anyone who promises results overnight or in a short period such as 1 week. As the chapter title suggests, it's consistency that is key in any fruitful endeavor, whether it's losing weight, gaining fitness, or building muscle.

Track your progress over time

As you won't see results immediately, they may happen so slowly that you don't notice them too much as you see yourself in the mirror daily. For this, you can either measure yourself using a tape measure in those trouble areas, or I would suggest taking pictures. For taking pictures and measuring I would recommend doing it under the same conditions. For example, if you took a picture after breakfast and you have a giant "food baby", then your belly may look oversized. The best time to weigh in, take pictures, or measure yourself, is first thing in the morning, (preferably after a bowel movement). This way you can keep a realistic track of your progress over time and you can view your progress, which will hopefully motivate you to keep going on, as you know what you're doing is working. If it's not working, then change it up! The definition of insanity is doing the same thing, over and over, and expecting a different result, DON'T be insane!

Be prepared to wait

The last thing I have to add here is, weight loss is often a waiting game, you sure as hell didn't gain all that weight overnight and you will no doubt take even more time to lose it. Be patient, enjoy the process, and know that you're doing the right thing. Even at times it may seem like you're getting nowhere or the progress is so slow that you can barely notice. I honestly think, if you follow and live by my ways in this book, then you'll be set up for life on a weight loss path. So don't worry about getting to your goal weight within a year or before the wedding, just focus on getting there and if it's not coming fast enough, if you're not already doing a lot of cardio, increase it. If you're not already eating as whole foods as possible, then eat that way. If you keep eating the correct way and exercising daily over a period of time, you WILL see results, I assure you. Just keep focused and don't let anything stop you!

Chapter 16 Conclusion

- Don't expect to see results overnight, these things take time.

- Track your progress over time so you can see the changes, whether it's with pictures or some kind of graph.

- Be prepared to wait, anything that is worth having, is worth waiting for.

- You didn't get fat overnight, and you won't get slim overnight either.

Chapter 17 – Conclusion

To sum up this book

In this chapter I thought that I'd sum up this book in a manageable and easy to read summary for re-reading in the future. Throughout this book, I've talked about how to change your mindset from the typical eat less, exercise more to weigh less mindset. I'm sure you've been there and done that. I really hope you can leave this book with all the information that you need to go out there and have a successful weight loss journey. The main reason I wrote this, is because I've seen far too many books out there promoting fads or unsustainable living. Whether it's low carb, low calorie, or a mixture of the two. I want to put some positive information out there which really works. I don't expect to become rich from this book, nor do I expect for it to make the New York Times best sellers list. This isn't because I don't have faith in either my writing ability or the information I've provided, but rather because I don't think the mainstream media is ready for this book, nor will they promote it, or maybe even not be allowed to? For many of you who are not accustomed to my alternative ideas behind weight loss, this book may have seemed strange and totally radical to you, but thank you for sticking with it up to this point.

Dieting, weighing in, and comparing yourself to others

Don't ever see what you're doing as a "diet", instead see it as a lifestyle which is sustainable for life, which it needs to be, in order to be successful long term. You don't want to end up like the biggest loser contestants, losing all that weight, but bouncing back and gaining the weight back, plus extra! Forget about what other people look like, you are not them, and will never look exactly like them, no matter how hard you try. Instead focus on looking like the greatest version of yourself, whatever shape or size that might be. Aspiring to celebrity bodies or physiques is often unattainable for us, because behind the scenes they are often using steroids or other secret weight loss aids to lose or gain weight for roles in a very short time period. Don't rely on the number on the scales day to day as it can fluctuate and vary from day to day, especially during times such as women's periods. Instead you can weigh yourself under the same conditions once a week, and keep a log of it and make sure the weight it falling over time. For example, you may lose 0.5lbs one week but 3lbs another week, so don't let it bother you. The main thing is to keep a picture record of yourself from month to month to make sure you're seeing the changes.

Eating for weight loss in a nutshell

Throughout this book, I've proposed many alternative ideas behind what our natural diet is, what we should and shouldn't eat. Here I want to outline these points into this chapter for reference. By nature, we are herbivores and our bodies are designed to eat those foods only. Our teeth, our nails, our intestine lengths, and our stomach acid, suggests we are NOT designed to eat meat. As for dairy, no other creature in nature drinks milk from another animal and no animal drinks milk upon adulthood. Eggs are also not a natural part of our diet, are not even considered healthy and not allowed to be referred to as such, as stated by the USDA. Eggs contain high amounts of saturated fat and cholesterol which is very unhealthy for our heart and cardiovascular system. Focus your diet on whole foods with the addition of refined sugars, the more natural and unprocessed, the better. Try to eat as many different colors of food as possible, as each color contains different nutrients. I post my almost daily meals on my Instagram channel so you can be sure to check that out for ideas and inspiration <u>here</u>

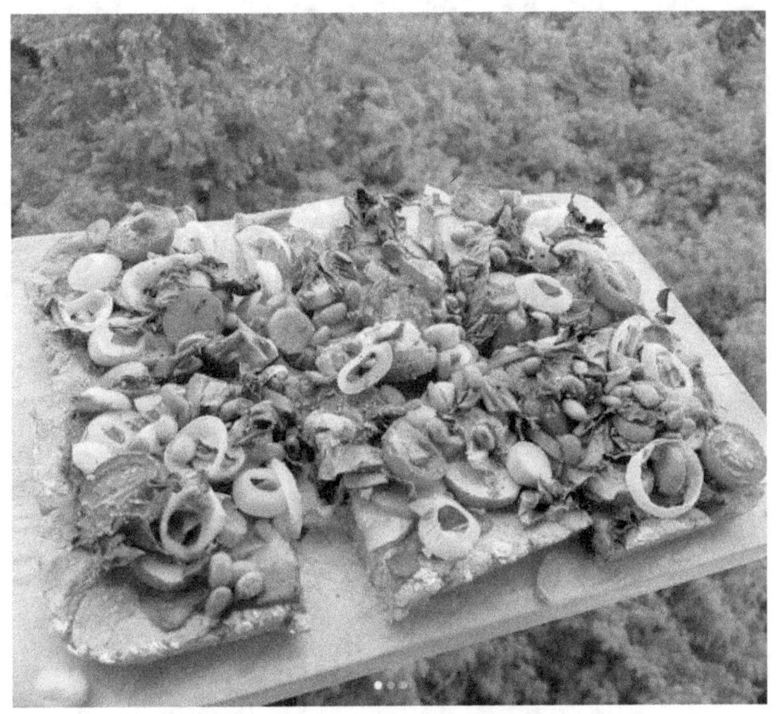

Sweet potato crust pizza with vegetables and beans.

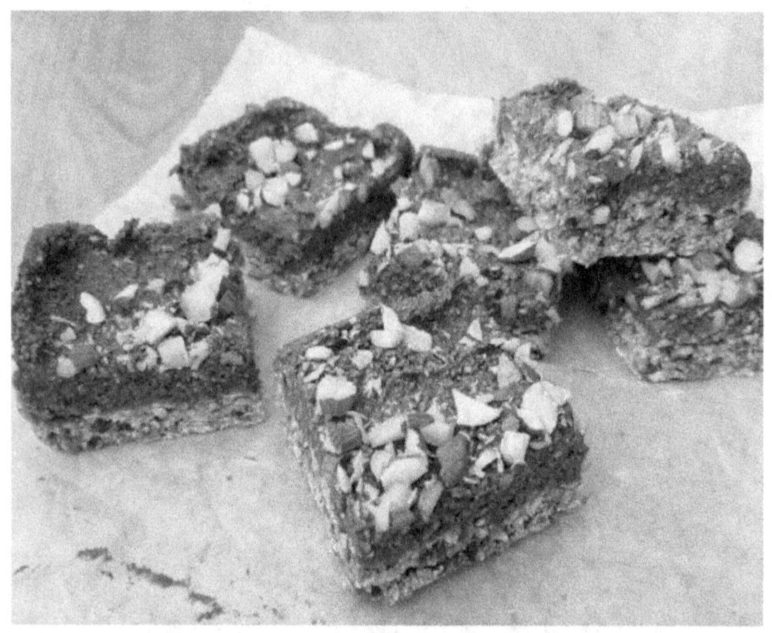

Chocolate and peanut butter oatmeal bars.

There are so many exciting recipes you can make, be sure to head to Instagram and YouTube for recipes and inspiration. You can search using tags like: #plantbased #whatveganseat #highcarb #wholefoods #carbthefuckup

You will never get bored of the variety and there is so many great ideas! Eat intuitively, don't stuff yourself beyond satiation, and don't leave a meal unsatisfied.

Loosing excuses and staying consistent

I could have written a book on these topics alone but I had to condense the topics as much as possible. Break the habit of making excuses to excuse yourself from getting stuff done, whether it's exercising or eating the right foods, lose the excuses and find your results! Remember that consistency is a fundamental part of achieving weight loss and a healthy lifestyle. Staying on track for 2 weeks and falling off for 2 weeks is a sure-fire way to never achieve true health.

Exercising for weight loss

Remember to remain consistent with any exercising endeavor and keep it sustainable. Stay in the low zones (1-2), the majority of the time, as that's where you will burn the greatest amount of fat in the long run. Although in zone 3 you burn *more* fat than zone 2, you also burn *more* glucose and you damage muscles quicker, leading to less total workload. Try to factor exercising into your daily life such as walking or cycling to work or to the shops instead of using your car or public transport where possible. Commuting to work can be an easy way to get anywhere from 5 hours to 10 hours of exercise in each week, without even having to "work out". Get out of the lazy mentality of taking the lift, when you can quite easily take the stairs.

Thanks again

Thank you so much for making it through this book, I really hope you've enjoyed it so far. I've tried to make the subjects light and easy to digest for people new to the whole weight loss scene. I hope you can get even a fraction of the results I got with the same information found inside this book. Thanks again for purchasing this book and I wish you the best luck on your weight loss journey! However long or short it may be. Just remember the information and put it into practice and I have no doubt you'll do well in any future weight loss or fitness endeavors.

If you need any further help or information, feel free to email me: cyclingslimmer@gmail.com

If you have trouble motivating yourself to take on the information found in this book and need some guidance or just someone to keep you accountable, then I offer one-on-one personal coaching, drop me an email for more info: cyclingslimmer@gmail.com

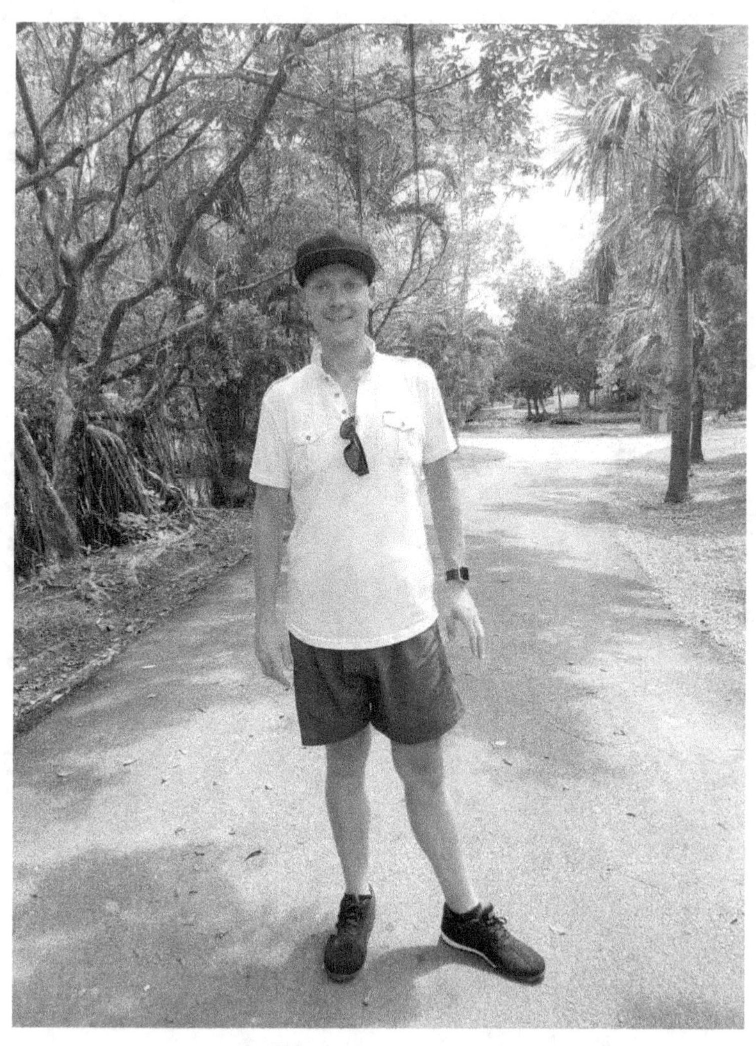

I wish you all the best, Craig Roberts.